PROGRESS IN CLINICAL AND BIOLOGICAL RESEARCH

Please contact the publisher for information about previous titles in this series.

ADVANCES IN CANCER CONTROL
The War on Cancer—
15 Years of Progress

ADVANCES IN CANCER CONTROL
The War on Cancer— 15 Years of Progress

Proceedings of the Fourth Annual Meeting on Advances in Cancer Control— A Combined Meeting of the Association of Community Cancer Centers/ Association of American Cancer Institutes, held in Washington, D.C., April 2–6, 1986

Editors

Paul F. Engstrom
Fox Chase Cancer Center
Philadelphia, Pennsylvania

Lee E. Mortenson
ELM Services, Inc.
Rockville, Maryland

Paul N. Anderson
Penrose Cancer Hospital
Colorado Springs, Colorado

ALAN R. LISS, INC. • NEW YORK

Address all Inquiries to the Publisher
Alan R. Liss, Inc., 41 East 11th Street, New York, NY 10003

Library of Congress Cataloging-in-Publication Data

Meeting on Advances in Cancer Control (4th : 1986 :
    Washington, D.C.)
    Advances in cancer control.

    (Progress in clinical and biological research ;
v. 248)
    Held in conjunction with the 12th National
Meeting of the Association of Community Cancer
Centers.
    Includes bibliographies and index.
    1. Cancer—Prevention—Congresses. I. Engstrom,
Paul F., 1936–   . II. Mortenson, Lee E.
III. Anderson, Paul N. IV. Association of
Community Cancer Centers. V. Association of
American Cancer Institutes. VI. Association of
Community Cancer Centers. Meeting (12th : 1986 :
Washington, D.C. VII. Title. VIII. Series.
[DNLM: 1. Neoplasms—prevention & control—
congresses.   Wl PR668E v.248 / QZ 200 M495 1986a]
RC268.M44   1986   616.99'405   87-16954
ISBN 0-8451-5098-7

Contents

Contributors

Zili Amsel, Fox Chase Cancer Center, Philadelphia, PA 19111 **[67,161,191]**

Paul N. Anderson, Penrose Cancer Hospital, Colorado Springs, CO **[xvii]**

Taka Ashikaga, Department of Biostatistics, University of Vermont, Burlington, VT 05405 **[27]**

Jan R. Atwood, College of Nursing, University of Arizona, Tucson, AZ 85724 **[263]**

Carey Azzara, Dana-Farber Cancer Institute, Boston, MA 02115 **[173]**

Andrew M. Balshem, Fox Chase Cancer Center, Philadelphia, PA 19111 **[161]**

Louis S. Beliczky, Department of Industrial Hygiene, United Rubber Workers International Union, Akron, OH 44308 **[75]**

Isak Berker, Lapeer General Hospital, Lapeer, MI 48446 **[229]**

D. Blayney, Wilshire Oncology Medical Group and Los Angeles Oncologic Institute, Los Angeles, CA 92057 **[299]**

A. Bouzaglou, Wilshire Oncology Medical Group and Los Angeles Oncologic Institute, Los Angeles, CA 92057 **[299]**

Bryce Breitenstein, Hanford Environmental Health Foundation, Richland, WA 99352 **[93]**

Debbie Butler, San Joaquin Valley Community Clinical Oncology Program, Fresno, CA 93715 **[217]**

Leslie A. Clegg, Department of Industrial Hygiene, United Rubber Workers International Union, Akron, OH 44308 **[75]**

J. P. Concannon, Division of Medical Oncology, Allegheny General Hospital and Allegheny Singer Research Institute, Pittsburgh, PA 15212; present address: Radiation Oncology, Beaver Medical Center, Beaver, PA, 15212 **[289]**

Michael C. Costanza, Department of Biostatistics, University of Vermont, Burlington, VT 05405 **[27]**

Susan Curry, Fred Hutchinson Cancer Research Center, Seattle, WA 98104 **[93]**

M. H. Dalbow, Division of Medical Oncology, Allegheny General Hospital and Allegheny Singer Research Institute, Pittsburgh, PA 15212 **[289]**

Sharon W. Davis, Fox Chase Cancer Center, Philadelphia, PA 19111 **[145]**

The numbers in brackets are the opening page numbers of the contributors' articles.

Hari H. Dayal, Epi-Stat Research Laboratory, Fox Chase Cancer Center, Philadelphia, PA and the Department of Preventive Medicine and Community Health, University of Texas Medical Branch, Galveston, TX **[245]**

J. Dolan, Wilshire Oncology Medical Group and Los Angeles Oncologic Institute, Los Angeles, CA 92057 **[299]**

Mark A. Donavan, Southwestern Vermont Medical Center, Bennington, VT **[213]**

Anne L. Dorwaldt, Office of Health Promotion Research, University of Vermont, Burlington, VT 05405 **[27]**

Gordon L. Doty, Providence Medical Center, Portland, OR 97213 **[53]**

Marilyn A. Driscoll, Department of Surgery and the Vermont Regional Cancer Center, University of Vermont, Burlington, VT 05405 **[27]**

Kate Duffy, Dana-Farber Cancer Institute, Boston, MA 02115 **[173]**

William M. Dugan, Jr., Cancer Center, Methodist Hospital of Indiana, Inc., Indianapolis, IN 46202 **[303]**

Morry Edwards, Borgess Mental Health Center, Borgess Medical Center, Kalamazoo, MI 49001 **[153]**

Robert E. Enck, Riverside Regional Cancer Institute, Riverside Methodist Hospital, Columbus, OH 43214 **[183]**

Paul F. Engstrom, Fox Chase Cancer Center, Philadelphia, PA 19111 **[xvii,67,123,135,145,161,191]**

Lorenz Finison, Dana-Farber Cancer Institute, Boston, MA 02115 **[173]**

Marshall S. Flam, San Joaquin Valley Community Clinical Oncology Program, Fresno, CA 93715 **[217]**

Linda Fleisher, Fox Chase Cancer Center, Philadelphia, PA 19111 **[135]**

Brian S. Flynn, Office of Health Promotion Research, University of Vermont, Burlington, VT 05405 **[27]**

Roger S. Foster, Jr., Department of Surgery and the Vermont Regional Cancer Center, University of Vermont, Burlington, VT 05405 **[27]**

Michael W. Fry, School of Pharmacy and Pharmacal Sciences, Purdue University, West Lafayette, IN 47907 **[303]**

K. Gala, Wilshire Oncology Medical Group and Los Angeles Oncologic Institute, Los Angeles, CA 92057 **[299]**

Dan George, Hurley Medical Center, Flint, MI 48502 **[233]**

Mary Lou Giddings, Rutland Regional Medical Center, Rutland, VT 05701 **[213]**

Doris Gillespie, Fox Chase Cancer Center, Philadelphia, PA 19111 **[161,191]**

Diane Gordon, Providence Medical Center, Portland, OR 97213 **[53]**

Ann Guidera-Matey, Fox Chase Cancer Center, Philadelphia, PA 19111 **[161]**

Neel Hammond, Billings Interhospital Oncology Project, Billings, MT **[205]**

Nancy Hessol, Hanford Environmental Health Foundation, Richland, WA 99352 **[93]**

E.E. Ho, Cancer Prevention and Control Program, Arizona Cancer Center, University of Arizona, Tucson, AZ 85724; present address: Adult Health Section, California Department of Health Services, Sacramento, CA 95814 **[263]**

Godfrey M. Hochbaum, Lineberger Cancer Research Center, University of North Carolina, Chapel Hill, NC 27514 **[75]**

J. Hughes, Kelsey-Seybold Foundation's Cancer Prevention Center, Houston, TX 77030 **[109]**

G. Jackson, Kelsey-Seybold Foundation's Cancer Prevention Center, Houston, TX 77030 **[109]**

L. Jund, Oncology Program, Queen of the Valley Hospital, West Covina, CA 91790 **[299]**

Arnold D. Kaluzny, Lineberger Cancer Research Center, University of North Carolina, Chapel Hill, NC 27514 **[75]**

Sandra Kampen, Billings Interhospital Oncology Project, Billings, MT **[205]**

Martha K. Keintz, Fox Chase Cancer Center, Philadelphia, PA 19111 **[123,135,191]**

P. Kennedy, Wilshire Oncology Medical Group and Los Angeles Oncologic Institute, Los Angeles, CA 92057 **[299]**

Linda Kratcha-Sveningson, Community Clinical Oncology Program, St. Luke's Hospitals/Fargo Clinic, Fargo, ND 58122 **[129]**

Michael J. Krueger, Department of Industrial Hygiene, United Rubber Workers International Union, Akron, OH 44308 **[75]**

DeAnn Lazovich, San Joaquin Valley Community Clinical Oncology Program, Fresno, CA 93715 **[217]**

Y. Y. Lee, Lineberger Cancer Research Center, University of North Carolina, Chapel Hill, NC 27514 **[75]**

Peter A. Levine, Greater Flint Area Hospital Assembly's CHOP, Flint, MI 48504 **[225,229,233]**

Michael Levy, Fox Chase Cancer Center, Philadelphia, PA 19111 **[123]**

Norma MacElwee, Fox Chase Cancer Center, Philadelphia, PA 19111 **[123]**

Elizabeth Mallon, Dana-Farber Cancer Institute, Boston, MA 02115 **[173]**

Ben Marchello, Billings Interhospital Oncology Project, Billings, MT **[205]**

Barbara A. McCann, Accreditation Program for Hospice Care and Joint Commission on Accreditation for Hospitals, Chicago, IL 60611 **[183]**

R. Sue McPherson, Department of Cancer Prevention and Control, The University of Texas M.D. Anderson Hospital and Tumor Institute, Houston, TX 77030 **[255]**

J. Melville, Wilshire Oncology Medical Group and Los Angeles Oncologic Institute, Los Angeles, CA 92057 **[299]**

Frank L. Meyskens, Jr., Cancer Prevention and Control Program, Arizona Cancer Center, University of Arizona, Tucson, AZ 85724 **[263]**

Marie Michnich, School of Public Health, University of Washington, Seattle, WA 98195 **[93]**

Anthony B. Miller, Department of Preventive Medicine and Biostatistics, University of Toronto, Toronto, Ontario, Canada **[9]**

M. Minkoff, Kelsey-Seybold Foundation's Cancer Prevention Center, Houston, TX 77030 **[109]**

Lee E. Mortenson, ELM Services, Inc., Rockville, MD **[xvii]**

Phyllis Ager Mowry, San Joaquin Valley Community Clinical Oncology Program, Fresno, CA 93715 **[217]**

Willys Mueller, Department of Pathology, Hurley Medical Center, Flint, MI 48502 **[225]**

David Myers, Billings Interhospital Oncology Project, Billings, MT **[205]**

L. Nathanson, Winthrop-University Hospital and Nassau Regional CCOP, Mineola, NY 11501 and SUNY at Stony Brook, Stony Brook, NY 11790 **[283]**

Guy R. Newell, Department of Cancer Prevention and Control, The University of Texas M.D. Anderson Hospital and Tumor Institute, Houston, TX 77030 **[255]**

Richard Nixon [3]

Susan Oehme, Dana-Farber Cancer Institute, Boston, MA 02115 **[173]**

Linda V. O'Halloran, Community Clinical Oncology Program, St. Luke's Hospitals/Fargo Clinic, Fargo, ND 58122 **[129]**

Gilbert Omenn, Fred Hutchinson Cancer Research Center, Seattle, WA 98104 and School of Public Health, University of Washington, Seattle, WA 98195 **[93]**

Peter J. Parashos, Cancer Center, Methodist Hospital of Indiana, Inc., Indianapolis, IN 46202 **[303]**

Electra Pasket, Cancer Prevention Research Unit W–202, Fred Hutchinson Cancer Research Center, Seattle, WA 98103 **[39]**

W. Bradford Patterson, Dana-Farber Cancer Institute, Boston, MA 02115 **[173]**

Arthur Peterson, Fred Hutchinson Cancer Research Center, Seattle, WA 98104 and School of Public Health, University of Washington, Seattle, WA 98195 **[93]**

C. A. Presant, Wilshire Oncology Medical Group and Los Angeles Oncologic Institute, Los Angeles, CA 92057 **[299]**

R. P. Pugh, Division of Medical Oncology, Allegheny General Hospital and Allegheny Singer Research Institute, Pittsburgh, PA 15212 **[289]**

R. N. Raju, Division of Medical Oncology, Allegheny General Hospital and Allegheny Singer Research Institute, Pittsburgh, PA 15212 **[289]**

Mildred A. Reardon, Medical Center Hospital of Vermont, Burlington, VT **[213]**

John A. Reinsch, San Joaquin Valley Community Clinical Oncology Program, Fresno, CA 93715 **[217]**

Thomas C. Ricketts, Lineberger Cancer Research Center, University of North Carolina, Chapel Hill, NC 27514 **[75]**

M. Rigas, Department of Pharmacy, Queen of the Valley Hospital, West Covina, CA 91790 **[299]**

Barbara Rimer, Fox Chase Cancer Center, Philadelphia, PA 19111 **[123,135,191]**

Bienvenido T. Samson, Fox Chase Cancer Center, Philadelphia, PA 19111 **[145]**

Anna P. Schenck, Lineberger Cancer Research Center, University of North Carolina, Chapel Hill, NC 27514 **[75]**

L. L. Schenken, Division of Medical Oncology, Allegheny General Hospital and Allegheny Singer Research Institute, Pittsburgh, PA 15212 **[289]**

J. Schindler, Department of Pharmacy, Queen of the Valley Hospital, West Covina, CA 91790 **[299]**

Mary Sexton, Department of Epidemiology, University of Maryland Medical School, Baltimore, MD 21201 **[93,101]**

Jan Sinsheimer, Fred Hutchinson Cancer Research Center, Seattle, WA 98104 **[101]**

Laura J. Solomon, Department of Psychology, University of Vermont, Burlington, VT 05405 **[27]**

Donna J. Stover, Kalamazoo Community Hospital Oncology Program, Kalamazoo, MI 49001 **[237]**

Rosalind P. Thomas, Lineberger Cancer Research Center, University of North Carolina, Chapel Hill, NC 27514 **[75]**

Beti Thompson, Cancer Prevention Research Unit W–202, Fred Hutchinson Cancer Research Center, Seattle, WA 98103 **[39,93,101]**

Nicole Urban, Cancer Prevention Research Unit W–202, Fred Hutchinson Cancer Research Center, Seattle, WA 98103 **[39]**

John Valentine, Central Vermont Hospital, Berlin, VT **[213]**

H. James Wallace, Jr., Rutland Regional Medical Center, Rutland, VT 05701 **[213]**

Michael J. Wargovich, Section of Gastrointestinal Oncology and Digestive Diseases, M.D. Anderson Hospital and Tumor Institute, University of Texas System Cancer Center, Houston, TX 77030 **[313]**

Nancy White, Borgess Medical Center, Kalamazoo, MI 49001 **[153]**

M. E. Williams, Winthrop-University Hospital and Nassau Regional CCOP, Mineola, NY 11501 and SUNY at Stony Brook, Stony Brook, NY 11790 **[283]**

Christine M. Wilson, Fox Chase Cancer Center, Philadelphia, PA 19111 **[135,145]**

C. Wiseman, Wilshire Oncology Medical Group and Los Angeles Oncologic Institute, Los Angeles, CA 92057 **[299]**

John K. Worden, Office of Health Promotion Research, University of Vermont, Burlington, VT 05405 **[27]**

Stephen W. Workman, Fox Chase Cancer Center, Philadelphia, PA 19111 **[67]**

C. F. Zamerilla, Division of Medical Oncology, Allegheny General Hospital and Allegheny Singer Research Institute, Pittsburgh, PA 15212 **[289]**

B. L. Zidar, Division of Medical Oncology, Allegheny General Hospital and Allegheny Singer Research Institute, Pittsburgh, PA 15212 **[289]**

L. Zimmerman, Kelsey-Seybold Foundation's Cancer Prevention Center, Houston, TX 77030 **[109]**

Introduction: Fifteen Years of Progress in Cancer Control

The fourth annual meeting of the Advances in Cancer Control held jointly by the Association of Community Cancer Centers and the Association of American Cancer Institutes occurred April 2–6, 1986 in Washington, D.C in conjunction with the 12th National Meeting of the Association of Community Cancer Centers. The day-long meeting started with a plenary session and a keynote address by Dr. Anthony Miller, Director of the Canadian Cancer Institute in Toronto, Canada. Dr. Miller addressed the feasibility of preventing cancers through changes in social habits such as smoking cessation and dietary habits, as well as the likelihood that screening technologies would reduce the impact of invasive cancer. Five scientific sessions were held through the day. The largest was a four-hour program devoted to abstracts on population-based cancer control chaired by Knut Ringen, Dr. P.H., the Division of Cancer Prevention and Control at the National Cancer Institute and Barbara Rimer, Dr.P.H., Director of Health Communication Research at the Fox Chase Cancer Center in Philadelphia. The second ACCC/AACI scientific session was on diet, nutrition, and chemo-prevention chaired by George L. Blackburn, M.D., Ph.D., Associate Professor of Surgery, Harvard Medical School and of the New England Deaconess Hospital in Boston, Massachusetts. Three other scientific sessions were sponsored by the ACCC; the session titles and the moderators were: 1) Administrative Trends, Marsha Jean Fountain, R.N., M.N., St. Joseph Cancer Center, Albuquerque, New Mexico; 2) Clinical Practice Trends, Lloyd K. Everson, M.D., Chief of Oncology, the Fargo Clinic and St. Luke's Hospitals, Fargo, North Dakota; and 3) Research in the Community, Irwin D. Fleming, M.D., President of the Medical Staff, Methodist Hospital of Memphis and Chief of Surgical Services, St. Jude's Children's Research Hospital, Memphis, Tennessee. In addition to presentations based on submitted abstracts, a poster session covering related topics was held in the evening. The highlight of the ACCC meeting was the address by former President Richard Nixon entitled, "The War Against Cancer."

In order to organize this volume of Advances in Cancer Control: Fifteen Years of Progress, the editors have placed the two keynote addresses at the beginning to underscore the importance of the National Cancer Act of 1971 and to place in perspective the progress made in the prevention and early detection of cancer. The submitted papers have been rearranged into four sections of equal size: Section I, Research on Selected Populations; Section II, Research on Cancer Control Interventions; Section III, Trends in Community Cancer Programs; and Section IV, Clinical and Epidemiological Research.

We note, with some degree of satisfaction that cancer control research and clinical research in community hospital settings have taken on a degree of sophistication that wasn't present in the initial conference on Advances in Cancer Control five years ago. Not only are more of the community physicians and health care providers active in the research programs, a number of the comprehensive cancer centers have also developed cancer control research programs that are producing results and affecting the way physicians and hospitals conduct cancer screening as well as cancer symptom control. The papers in Section I, Research in Selected Populations include studies of breast cancer screening, colorectal cancer screening and multisite screening in community settings, and a series of papers on worksite cancer control, especially as it related to smoking cessation projects. The papers in Section II on Cancer Control Interventions include studies on pain control, a survey of chemotherapy handlers relative to their health risks, impact of a cancer program for older people, a cancer patients' survey on psychosocial needs and evaluation of hospice care. Trends in community cancer programs include a discussion of four community cooperative oncology programs (CCOP's), as well as an analysis of the impact on referrals, competition and organization of collaborative health care programs in the communities. The clinical and epidemiological research studies are well designed and look at cancer risk vs. socioeconomic status and race, the use of food frequency techniques in nutritional research, the application of new chemotherapy programs or intravenous antiemetic programs in cancer patients, a study of circulating marker in ovarian cancer and the search for new cancer chemoprevention agents.

This issue of Advances in Cancer Control: Fifteen Years of Progress will further stimulate cancer control investigators, community oncologists, and hospital and health administrators who are faced with new and challenging cancer control issues in the 1980's. They have made the most of the opportunity given them through the National Cancer Act of 1971.

Paul F. Engstrom
Lee E. Mortenson
Paul N. Anderson

KEYNOTE ADDRESSES

Advances in Cancer Control: The War on Cancer—
15 Years of Progress, pages 3–8
© 1987 Alan R. Liss, Inc.

THE WAR AGAINST CANCER

Address by Former President Richard Nixon Upon
Accepting the Award for Service to Cancer Patients
of the Association of Community Cancer Centers

In expressing my appreciation of this award, may I in turn
thank the members of this organization for what you have
contributed to the cause of cancer prevention and treatment.
The 300 community cancer centers you represent manage twenty-
five percent of all cancer cases in the United States. You
are the front line troops in the war against cancer. All
Americans are in your debt.

When I signed The National Cancer Act two days before
Christmas in 1971, I said: "I hope in the years ahead we will
look back on this action today as the most significant action
taken during this Administration."

How could I say that-particularly in view of what had
happened just in the year 1971? On July 15 I had announced
my trip to China, which led to an historic new relationship
between China and the United States. In October, I had
announced my trip to Moscow, which led to the first Soviet-
U.S. nuclear arms limitation agreements. By the end of that
year, we had reduced our forces and casualties in Vietnam by
seventy-five percent. All of these actions were major steps
toward a more peaceful world. How could a new cancer
initiative compare with them in importance?

Let me answer that question on two levels-strategic and
personal. From a strategic standpoint, we must recognize
that more Americans die each year from cancer than were
killed in action in all four years of World War II.

From a personal standpoint, there were several reasons for my deep commitment to the cause of finding a cure for cancer.

When Mrs. Nixon was only twelve years old her mother died of cancer.

When I was in high school, one of my favorite aunts, to whom I was deeply attached, died of cancer.

There were three incidents while I was Vice President that seared my memory. Early in 1953 I spoke to the President's Business Advisory Council in Hot Spring, Virginia. Senator Robert Taft preceded me on the program. He made some uncharacteristically rude remarks about businessmen in general which shocked those in the audience, most of whom were his friends. When he completed his remarks, he abruptly got up and left the room pushing his wife, Martha, ahead of him in her wheelchair. I notice that he limped as he walked. I turned to the chairman and said, "Ignore his comments. I sense that he just isn't feeling well." Two months later he died of cancer.

I shall never forget the last time I saw John Foster Dulles on May 20, 1959. I often visited him at Walter Reed Hospital where he was terminally ill with cancer. As the nurse wheeled him into the reception room that day, I noted that he was painfully thin. His voice was weaker than usual. But his superb mind had become even sharper as his physical condition deteriorated.

When I visited him, he never talked about his physical problems. He always preferred to discuss the great foreign policy issues to which he had devoted his life. On this occasion, I asked him what advice he had for me for my meeting with Khrushchev, which was to take place the following month. I told him that some Soviet experts in the media were insisting that my major goal should be to convince Khrushchev that the United States did not threaten him and that we were sincerely for peace. He disagreed. He said, "Khrushchev does not need to be convinced of our good intentions. He knows we don't threaten him. He understands us. What he needs to know is that we understand him. Rather than trying to convince him that we are for peace, you should try to convince him that he cannot win a war." It was the best advice I ever received on Soviet-American relations. Four days later he died.

My most vivid recollection is of a day that I was presiding over the Senate. The regular chaplain was out of town and a visiting chaplain gave the invocation. I always listened to the invocation because more often that not it was the best speech of the day-which may be damning it with faint praise. Afterwards, I shook hands with him and he asked me if I could give him an autograph for his daughter who, as I recall, was eight years old, the same age as my daughter Julie. He told me she was an only child. His wife and he had always wanted children, and when this little girl was born after fifteen years of marriage he said she was like a gift from heaven. I asked where she went to school. He told me that she was no longer able to go to school; she was in the National Health Institute being treated for leukemia. That afternoon Gina Lollobrigida made a courtesy call on me in my Capitol office and presented me with two beautiful Italian walking dolls for my two daughters, Tricia and Julie. That night I told them about the dolls and the little girl in the hospital. They wanted to keep the dolls, but they urged me to give them to her.

The next day at the National Health Institute, I had one of the most rewarding conversations of my life with the little girl and her roommate, who was also suffering from leukemia. I went there to cheer them up. Their liveliness and irrepressible spirit cheered me up.

A few months later, I learned that the little girl had died holding the Italian doll in her arms.

What progress has been made in the fifteen years since the national cancer initiative? The federal budget for cancer programs has increased from $230 million in 1971 to 1.25 billion in 1985. Contributions to the American Cancer Society have increased from $70 million in 1971 to $240 million in 1985. The number of medical oncologist-cancer specialists has increased from 100 in 1970 to over 2,800 in 1980. There were only three comprehensive cancer centers in the United States in 1971; there are over 20 today.

But what are the results of all of this additional money and effort? First, the bad news: We have learned that unlike polio or tuberculosis, there is no one cure for cancer. There are many different kinds of cancer. Cancer is a

Hydraheaded monster. The death rate from cancer is still
increasing. Four hundred seventy-two thousand people will
die from cancer this year-an increase of ten thousand over
last year.

But now for the good news: While there is no one cure for
cancer, cures have been found for some types of cancer. In
1971, there were cures for only two types of cancer in cases
where it had spread from the point of origin. Today, there
are cures for twelve types of cancer which have spread from
the point of origin. While the death rate from cancer has
moderately increased, the survival rate of those diagnoed and
treated for cancer has increased dramatically.

Most striking is that the survival rate for children with
cancer has increased from ten percent in 1970 to over fifty
percent in 1985. Among all cancer patients in 1970, only
forty percent could hope to survive for five years or more
after treatment. Today, over fifty percent will survive.
Here are some examples comparing 1970 and 1983. The survival
rate for colon cancer has increased from forty-nine percent
to fifty-three percent, leukemia from twenty-two percent to
forty percent, breast cancer from sixty-eight percent to
seventy-five percent, prostate from sixty-three percent to
seventy-two percent, and Hodgkin's disease from sixty-seven
percent to seventy-three percent.

But statistics are too cold and impersonal to make the point.
Let me put it in personal terms. Two years ago I was deeply
distressed to learn that my brother Don, who is two years
younger than I, had a very severe case of Hodgkin's disease.
He has had a very rough time over the past two years going
through chemotherapy and other treatment. I saw him when I
was in California three weeks ago. He looked thin and weak
but his spirit was strong. He told me his doctor had told
him that if he had had only the treatment available fifteen
years ago, he would not be alive today.

One of the greatest advances in the past fifteen years is in
cancer prevention by early diagnosis and treatment. I recall
a meeting of the National Security Council early in 1953.
Seated at Eisenhower's right was General Hoyt Vandenberg, the
Air Force Chief of Staff. He was one of the most handsome
men in the service and a legendary World War II hero. A
great future lay before him. I noticed that he looked thin

and drawn as he briefed the President and members of the
Security Council on our Air Force capabilities. A few months
after that meeting, he died of cancer of the prostate.

Eisenhower's military aid, General Jerry Persons, was one of
Vandenberg's closest friends. He was deeply shocked because
he felt his death was so unnecessry. Vandenberg had not
found tho timo during his wartime service to have his routine
annual physicals which would have disclosed the problem and
cured it with a simple operation. In this audience today is
my former secretary, Rose Mary Woods. Just before Christmas
she was not feeling well. Her doctor insisted on a complete
physical. She was shocked when he diagnosed lung cancer-
particularly because she never smoked in her life. She has
had a difficult time after her operation, but the prognosis
is good. Had the doctor not insisted on the examination and
operation, she might not be here today.

Finally, there have been some encouraging developments in
basic research. Scientists have long believed that cancer
was caused by damage to certain genes. Since the passage of
the National Cancer Act, investigators at several
laboratories across the United States have identified for the
first time what are called oncogenes. They have begun to
learn how genes are damaged by certain chemicals ad how
cancer genes are activated. They have not yet found a cure,
but the first step in finding a cure is to find the cause and
they have made significant progress in that area.

We had high hopes when we launched this initiative fifteen
years ago that we would find a complete cure for cancer. We
have been disappointed in that respect, but we have made
significant progress on prevention and treatment. As Doctor
Yarbro has pointed out in his introductory remarks, over four
million Americans who are destined to get cancer will be
cured because of the new technology developed under the
National Cancer Act of 1971. The day is near when basic
cancer research will achieve a dramatic breakthrough.

When I visited China in 1972, Marshall Ye, a revered eighty-
year-old Chinese leader who had accompanied Mao and Chou En-
lai on the Long March escorted me to the Great Wall. In the
two hours we were in the car together, his primary interest
was not in the new U.S./Chinese strategic relationship but
the progress we were making in cancer research under the
initiative which I had announced in 1971. He observed that
the Chinese smoked too much and that lung cancer was sharply

increasing. I told him that I hoped one of the results of
our new relationship would be a program of cooperation
between Chinese and American doctors and scientists in cancer
and other medical research.

Four years later when I visited China again, I think I may
have discovered one of the reasons for his interest in our
cancer program. Premier Chou En-lai, my host, was too ill to
see me. He died of cancer a few weeks later.

Today the United States' political differences with the
Soviet Union are particularly great. Some will never be
settled due to the fact that our interests and theirs are
diametrically opposed. But we have one common interest which
should override all political differences. The United States
and the Soviet Union should be allies in the war against
disease and particularly against cancer, where Soviet death
rates are sharply up.

I believe American scientists and doctors are the best in the
world. We win more Nobel Prizes than any other country. But
we have no monopoly on wisdom. Great medical discoveries are
not limited by national boundaries They should never be
limited by national differences. We are waging the war
against cancer not just for ourselves alone but for all
mankind.

Thirteen years from now we will be celebrating the beginning
of a new year, the beginning of a new century, and the
beginning of a new millenium. It is a day which comes only
once in a thousand years. The twentieth century has been the
bloodiest century in history. One hundred forty million
people were killed in wars in this century. That is more
than all the people killed in wars in all of recorded history
before this century began.

But there have been some great positive developments as well
in the twentieth cenury. We have seen the automobile replace
the horse. We have learned to fly. We have split the atom.
We have developed radio, motion pictures, and television. We
have ushered in the age of computers. On the health front,
we have found cures for polio, tuberculosis, and other dread
diseases.

Before this century ends, the conquest of cancer could be our
greatest victory.

Advances in Cancer Control: The War on Cancer—
15 Years of Progress, pages 9–23
© 1987 Alan R. Liss, Inc.

APPROACHES TO CANCER CONTROL IN CANADA, AND INTERNATIONALLY

Anthony B. Miller, M.B., FRCP(C)

Department of Preventive Medicine
and Biostatistics
University of Toronto

INTRODUCTION

In this presentation I shall review the present status
of cancer control in Canada and also refer to various cancer
control considerations that are relevant internationally.
I shall base my comments on the international situation in
relation to a four month period I spent at the International
Agency for Research on Cancer (IARC) in Lyon last year. My
main task was to coordinate the production of a report on
"Cancer Causes, Occurrence and Control" which it is expected
will be released by the IARC by about the end of this year.
This is intended as advice to member governments of the
World Health organization on the steps they should be taking,
based on current knowledge, towards achieving cancer control
by the year 2000. The IARC report is still in draft and
anything I say in this presentation should not be regarded
as official policy of the IARC. Rather it is my own view
point after having this experience reviewing the international scene.

We are all aware that cancer control covers the whole
spectrum from primary prevention through to rehabilitation,
but today I shall be referring primarily to knowledge
relating to primary prevention and secondary prevention, or
screening. I shall refer only briefly to the possible
contribution of treatment and not at all to the problems of
rehabilitation.

TRENDS OF CANCER INCIDENCE IN MORTALITY

In Canada, as in the United States, the major increase in lung cancer in males has been largely responsible for the fact that both cancer incidence and mortality in males has been slowly rising for the last 40 years. In females in spite of a recent steep increase in incidence of lung cancer, overall cancer incidence and mortality has been falling. In Canada, as in the United States, in the 1930's stomach cancer was the commonest cancer in men, breast cancer in women. In the 1980's lung cancer is by far the commonest cancer in men, breast cancer is still the commonest in women but lung cancer will become a more important cause of cancer death than breast cancer in women by the end of this decade. Since about 1970, first in women and then in men, mortality from cancer of the large intestine has been falling. Although cancer registry data suggests an increase in incidence of large intestinal cancer, when the registry data are corrected for second primary tumors, it is apparent that incidence is also falling.

In the world generally the incidence of cancer is increasing dramatically. There are now more cancers diagnosed each year in the developing countries than in the developed and this disparity will increase by the year 2000. At that stage, even on the basis of population projections taking note of the aging of the population but using current incidence rates, it seems likely that there will be more than 10 million cancers a year diagnosed in the world.

THE CAUSES OF CANCER

In their review for the United States Doll and Peto[1] made estimates of the proportion of cancers attributable to various factors. I have attempted a similar exercise for Canada,[2] the table below sets out my conclusions.

Causes of Cancer Cases (%)

Diet	27%	Parity	5%
Sunlight	19%	Sexual Activity	4%
Tobacco	16%	Alcohol	4%
Family History	10%	Drugs	2%
Occupation	6%	Radiation	1%

This table emphasizes that when calculations are based on cancer incidence, because skin cancer is such an important cancer, sunlight takes on an important causative role. If we had based the table on causes of cancer deaths, diet would have increased to 30%, tobacco to 26%, occupation to 9% and sunlight would have fallen to just 1%.

Although I would not like to minimize the importance of control of cancer through protection against sunlight, or the importance of controlling occupational causes of cancer when they are identified, in terms of the general public I believe that most attention needs to be paid to primary prevention through modification of diet and control of tobacco. I shall, therefore, concentrate on these two factors in the next two sections.

DIET ASSOCIATED CANCERS

Although currently there is no federal or provincial government policy with relation to primary prevention of cancer through diet modification, the Canadian Cancer Society, like the American Cancer Society has largely built upon the recommendations of the committee on Diet, Nutrition and Cancer of the National Research Council.[3] I believe the interim dietary guidelines of this committee have largely been sustained by the information that has accumulated since the report appeared and that they still form the basis of appropriate recommendations for the public. The guidelines proposed that in the North American diet fat consumption should be reduced from its present level of around 40% of calories to 30%, that green-yellow, cruciferous (brassica) vegetables and citrus fruits should be an important component of the daily diet, that salt cured, pickled and highly spiced foods should be avoided as far as possible and that alcohol should be drunk in moderation. To this both cancer societies of North America have added recommending the maintenance of ideal body weight which can be coupled with recommendations to avoid over-nutrition and caloric excess.

Direct evidence in support of these guidelines has been obtained in Canada for the three most important diet associated cancers, stomach, colo-rectum and breast. For stomach cancer our studies suggested that nitrite was the most important risk factor and that dietary fiber the most important protective factor.[4] It is not clear whether the protection stemmed from dietary fiber or from vitamin C intimately associated with fiber sources. Nevertheless, calculations based on our data suggested that it should be possible to prevent at least 80% of gastric cancer.

For colo-rectal cancer the most important risk factor was saturated fat intake with a dose-response relationship.[5] Analyses in relation to individual food items confirmed this for colon cancer though there was some suggestion for rectal cancer that some meats had an independent effect in increasing risk.[6] We could not demonstrate a protective effect of dietary fiber. Saxon Graham and his group had earlier suggested that vegetables of the brassica genus were protective,[7] fitting in with the observations of Wattenberg.[8] We were only able to find a weak protective effect of cruciferous vegetables after taking into consideration saturated fat intake. Recently it has been suggested that caloric intake may be more important than fat and that exercise may be protective.[9] A re-analysis of our data controlling for the effect of higher caloric intake in the cases than the controls still confirmed the overwhelming importance of saturated fat intake.[10] Indeed, this analysis suggested that rather than the proportional contribution of fat it is the absolute intake of fat that may be critical. Thus, possibly instead of advising both men and women to reduce fat consumption to 30% of calories or less, one should advise men to eat no more than 75 grams of fat daily and women no more than 50 grams. Calculations on the basis of our data suggest that at least 50% of colo-rectal cancer should be preventable by dietary modification.

Recently, Bruce and his colleagues from the Ludwig Institute in Toronto have proposed a hypothesis that the important variable may be the presence or absence of ionized calcium in the intestine at the time that fat is consumed.[11] Calcium is hypothesised to counteract the effect of free fatty acids and fecal bile acids in inducing loss of cells from the colonic epithelium, with subsequent proliferation and possible promotion of colo-rectal cancer. It has been proposed that this hypothesis should be tested in a chemo-prevention trial involving prescription of dietary calcium. Discussions are currently ongoing in Canada over such a trial.

Our first dietary study related to diet and breast cancer.[12] We found an association with total dietary fat intake but at that time no dose response relationship. A subsequent reanalysis using more modern approaches however identified saturated fat as the most important risk factor particularly in pre-menopausal women.[13] Two further studies in Canada have supported the association of fat and breast cancer.[14,15] Neither were able to take note of all sources of dietary fat, both found fat associated foods seemed to increase risk. Hislop's study suggested also that those who consumed fat on meat as a child also had increased risk.[15]

In addition to control of dietary fat it seems likely that reduction in obesity will reduce the risk of post-menopausal breast cancer and also possibly the risk of death in women who have breast cancer. A recent study from Israel shows a very strong relationship apparently independent of a dietary fat effect.[16]

We have calculated that at least 25% of breast cancer is attributable to dietary fat intake and 12% to obesity. The estimates in relation to dietary fat are almost certainly underestimates as both migrant studies and studies of special religious groups who have changed their diet to low or absent meat would suggest that the effect of diet on breast cancer has to operate early in life.[17] Our dietary studies are measuring current diet which may be a pale reflection of diet at the operative time period. Hence, we may be severely underestimating the contribution of fat reduction to eventual prevention of breast cancer.

A few small intervention trials are ongoing in Canada of agents such as beta-carotene, retinol, vitamin C and tocopherol using intermediate endpoints such as adenomatous polyps of the colon. There are also pilot studies evaluating the effect of low fat and high fiber diet on intermediate endpoints. So far we do not have any major large scale dietary intervention trials ongoing in Canada. Indeed, the most efficient way to proceed currently may be to make appropriate recommendations to the public and then carefully monitor subsequent trends in cancer incidence and mortality.

SMOKING ASSOCIATED CANCERS

Clearly the most important smoking associated cancer is lung cancer.[1] We know that the risk of lung cancer is proportional to the dose as well as the age at starting smoking. The higher the dose and the earlier the age the greater the lifetime risk. We also know that when people stop smoking their risk remains approximately at the same level and only appears to fall relative to continuing smokers. We also know that quitters are self-selected and that heavy smokers tend not to quit, so that possibly the best hope for control of smoking associated diseases is to prevent people starting or if they have started to get them to stop as soon as possible. Calculations of population attributable risks suggest that at least 80% of lung cancer in males is attributable to smoking and 45% to 80% in females with the proportion clearly increasing. Occupational factors also increase risk, particularly in males, with a population attributable risk of the order of 10% to 30%. Some studies have suggested that dietary factors may be protective.

Of other smoking associated cancers perhaps the most important is bladder cancer. Most studies have suggested a population attributable risk of smoking of around 50% in males and 25% in females.[18] Occupational factors are also clearly relevant in the causation of this cancer and dietary factors may be relevant. The other smoking associated cancers include pancreatic cancer, renal cancer, oral, esophageal and larynx cancer. For pancreatic cancer, the population attributable risk for smoking was of the order of 15% to 45% in males and 14% to 25% in females in various studies. Oral, esophageal and larynx cancer in a number of studies showed an interaction between smoking and alcohol. In many studies the interaction appears to be multiplicative so that full control of all these sites will only be achieved by control of both alcohol and smoking. In the west, alcohol seems to be more important than smoking for esophageal cancer, of equal importance to alcohol with oral cancer and possibly less important for laryngeal cancer. In the developing world chewing habits are important in the etiology of oral cancer, particularly in places like India with the chewing of betel nut with tobacco. Snuff dipping is increasing the risk of this cancer, particularly in parts of the United States.[19] Esophageal cancer is Asia and particularly in China does not seem to be related to the use of alcohol and tobacco, here dietary factors, as yet unidentified, may be important.[20]

Canada has been a participant in the endeavors of the International Union Against Cancer to promote control of smoking. The UICC have urged changing the behavior of the smoker and the potential smoker, changing the nature of the cigarette smoked towards a less harmful cigarette, changing the cultural background of society towards smoking and changing the economic and legislative climate towards smoking.[21] The Canadian Cancer Society has been active in public information and recently a number of municipal governments have moved with public opinion to control smoking in public places. The Federal government has done little towards a smoke-free environment especially at work and to this end voluntary agencies and government departments appear to be collaborating well.

In developing countries one of the major problems is the increase in prevalence of cigarette smoking aided by the advertising campaigns of multinational tobacco companies. The economic attractions of tobacco as a cash crop and a source of revenue to governments are competing with health objectives. It is clear if action is not taken soon, that just at the time we appear to be controlling our own epidemic in men, the epidemic of lung cancer in men in the developing countries will be getting into its stride.

SECONDARY PREVENTION (SCREENING)

The last decade has seen a gradual recognition of the fact that screening is expensive of health care resources and that unless demonstrated to be effective in the general population it cannot be regarded an an appropriate mechanism for cancer control.[22]

In Canada there have been two reports of a National Task Force evaluating screening for cancer of the cervix. The first concluded, as have others, that screening for cancer of the cervix is effective in reducing mortality from the disease.[23] It went on to make various recommendations in relation to quality control in laboratories and suggested that it was no longer necessary for women who were demonstrated to have had negative smears to continue an annual cervical smear throughout life. The second

reported at a time when concern was mounting that incidence
of cancer of the cervix might be increasing in young
women.[24] Such an increase has been noted in many countries
and would appear to be related to changes in sexual
practices in the young. Because insufficient knowledge was
available on the natural history of cancer of the cervix in
high risk groups, the Task Force decided to play safe and
recommended that women who have had sexual intercourse
should have screening annually from age 18 to 35 but congruent with their previous recommendation, at five year
intervals from age 35 to 60. Women over age 60 who had had
repeated satisfactory smears without significant atypia may
be dropped from a screening program. High priority should
be given to encouraging women at risk who have never had a
cervical cytology examination to have one.

The Task Force emphasized that a cervical cytology
screening program must have good organization. It recommended that all screening programs should have followup
systems to ensure that women with normal tests are recalled
at regular intervals for repeat testing, that action is
taken following discovery of an abnormality and that long
term followup is provided for patients treated for an
abnormality. They recommended the establishment of centralized regional or provincial registries across the country.
Although this recommendation has largely been ignored in
most areas of the country, the UICC group have recently
reinforced this, recommending that such registration should
be extended to identify all at risk women in the population
who should be specifically invited to attend for cervical
cytology screening. Only by such an organized system can
it be expected that the disease would eventually be fully
controlled.[25]

In the last decade mortality from cancer of the cervix
continued to decline in Canada though there has been a
suggestion that it may be increasing in women under the age
of 35.

The controversy over the frequency with which repeat
screening should be performed in women has raged both in
Canada and the United States. One way to approach this
problem directly is to assess the frequency of recurrence of
disease in women who have been recorded as having at least
one negative smear. Few programs have sufficient data to
assess the incidence of cancer of the cervix in women who

have been screened negative but by combining data from a number of programs in Canada and Europe the International Agency for Research on Cancer has been able to evaluate this directly.[26] It turns out that the protection from a single negative smear continues for about 5 years with some degree of protection thereafter. The study suggests that although maximum reduction in incidence of cancer of the cervix would follow annual screening from ages 20 to 64, screening every 3 years over the same age span results in over 90% reduction in incidence with less than half the number of tests a lifetime. Starting at age 26 would give almost as much protection while 5 yearly screening over the same age span would result in over 80% reduction in incidence, even 5 yearly screening from the ages of 35 to 64 involving only 6 tests a lifetime would result in 70% reduction in incidence.

It is already clear that cancer of cervix is very much more frequent in developing countries than in developed and the disparity will increase by the year 2000, when we expect a little over 100,000 cases to be diagnosed each year in the west but nearly 600,000 in the east. Screening for cancer of the cervix would place a major drain on health care resources in many developing countries which at the moment cannot afford the types of programs we are used to. A WHO working group has recommended that countries that can should aim to screen women at least once during the ages 35 to 40. Once they can afford more they should increase frequency of screening to every 10 years from age 35 to 55 and then every 5 years over the same age span. Only when resources become much more available would it be appropriate to extend screening down to the age of 25 and screen every three years.[27] These types of schedules have been designed to secure maximum impact at the ages of maximum incidence of cancer of the cervix.

Screening for breast cancer is the other major plank of cancer control based on screening. There is now possibly more information available on the effectiveness of screening for breast cancer derived from randomized trials and other types of study than for any other cancer. Nevertheless, there is still room for controversy over the effectiveness of screening for breast cancer at ages 40-49 and the relative contribution of mammography over and above physical examination. Both aspects are currently being investigated in a randomized controlled trial in Canada based on 15 centers

across the country with recruitment of just under 90,000
women starting in 1980 and being completed in 1985.[28]
Screening will cease in 1988 but it is still some years
before we can expect mortality results. In the meantime
we have confirmed information from other studies which
indicates the importance of quality control over mammography.[29] Careful attention has to be paid to technique:
mammography requires a dedicated unit with efficient
processing of films, accurate positioning of the patient
and firm compression of the breast. Attention has to be
paid to dosimetry with careful repeated monitoring to
ensure the best quality images at the lowest possible
radiation dose. A number of lesions are identified on
breast cancer screening ranging from cysts and mammary
dysplasia through benign atypical hyperplasia, borderline
abnormalities, insitu carcinomas with micro invasion
through to small invasive cancers. The use of mammography
has a number of effects on the community. Efficient locali-
zation, diagnoses and management of identified abnormalities
is required, this requires not only specimen radiography but
skilled radiologists, surgeons and pathologists. The
difficulties over this have recently been emphasized.[30] In
the National Breast Screening Study we have found that a
policy of screening based on physical examination resulted
in a benign to a malignant ratio in the first year of 3.5
falling to 1.8 in year 2. When mammography is added to
physical examination the ratio increases to 5.9 and 4.6
respectively.

Although the American Cancer Society and the American
College of Radiology have made a series of recommendations
over screening for breast cancer, there has been reluctance
to introduce a policy for screening for breast cancer in
Canada and indeed in many other countries. Part of the
difficulty relates to problems with patient management as
indicated, lack of radiologists and the lack of mammographic machines. Special training programs may have to be
introduced. Further, if mammography has little to add to
skilled physical examination of the breast in terms of
reduction in mortality then it may be more efficient to
base a screening program on specially trained examiners
such as nurses who have proven to be very efficient in our
National Breast Screening Study. Possible policies for
breast cancer screening based on present evidence would be
to offer screening only to women age 50 to 74 and to choose
between mammography with or without physical examination

given every two years compared to physical examination alone with mammography reserved for diagnosis probably given annually. In my view there is insufficient evidence yet available to advocate screening women under the age of 50.

Although there has been considerable interest in screening programs for colo-rectal cancer, so far other than a few pilot studies these have not been introduced in Canada. There are a number of problems over screening for this disease. One is dealing with a more elderly age group. Sigmoidoscopy has proven relatively unacceptable both to patient and to physicians. It is not yet clear whether flexible sigmoidoscopy will prove to be more acceptable. There is the difficulty over sensitivity of the occult blood test both in terms of possible precursors for cancer as well as cancers themselves. Occult blood tests especially with rehydration have been shown to be of low specificity which increases cost and introduces risk. Further, in spite of there having been two large studies ongoing in the United states, there has so far been no demonstrated mortality reduction.[31]

It has to be recognized that there are several obstacles to a major contribution of screening to cancer control. The natural history of the disease may not be amenable to secondary prevention. This appears to be applicable as far as lung cancer is concerned. There may have been poor evaluation of screening potential. It is important to recognize that case finding is not equivalent to mortality reduction. This may be a problem of screening for cancer of the colon and rectum currently. Poor organization has plagued many screening programs, particularly important in relation to screening for cancer of the cervix. There is the high cost of many screening tests, a particular problem now for mammography in many parts of the United States. There has been poor compliance of those at risk for disease, particularly in terms of screening for cancer of the cervix and there has been cost and morbidity from management of false positives, especially in terms of screening for cancer of the colon and rectum. Finally, there may have been over treatment of true positives. The too ready acceptance that an abnormality labelled as cancer must be treated early may have led to far too many biopsies or procedures performed for cancer of the breast.

It seems likely that only screening for cancer of the cervix and cancer of the breast carries an important potential for reduction in mortality following screening at the year 2000. It should be possible to reduce mortality from cancer of the cervix by at least 60% and from cancer of the breast on the basis of current knowledge, by about 25%. There is no potential contribution of screening to reduction in mortality from cancer of the lung and a possible but as of yet unestablished potential in relation to screening for cancers of the colon or rectum, for oral cancer, a problem particularly in developing countries, for cancer of the bladder, for cancer of the stomach currently being evaluated but with no confirmation of effectiveness in Japan and for cancer of the ovary.

CONCLUSIONS

It is important to recognize, when considering the potential impact of primary prevention, that there may be a long time scale before an appreciable impact can be detected in the population. This will be partly because of difficulties in pursuading people to change their habits if they have to take action but also because in the case of many primary preventive maneuvers they may have to operate early in life for maximum impact. Thus reduction in smoking, chewing or alcohol use could take at least five years to see any impact of any action and 40 years for maximum effectiveness. Vaccination against hepatitis B-virus, an important maneuver for primary prevention of liver cancer in developing countries, will take at least 30 years before any effect begins as vaccination has to be given in infancy and up to 60 years before a major effect can be expected. Changes in diet and nutrition carry some hope for a fairly early impact, say within five years in terms of cancer of the colon and rectum. But for other sites, particularly cancers of the breast and stomach, there may be 60 years before an important impact is seen. Reduction in obesity, important for post-menopausal breast cancer and for endometrial cancer, might show an effect within five years but a major impact would take twenty. Only for screening and any improvements in therapy is there much hope for an important impact within about ten years.

There is much interest currently in developing objectives for cancer control by the year 2000. Given our knowledge on the timing of the potential impact of preventive maneuvers it can be concluded that in terms of primary prevention the year 2000 impact will be small. However, there is no excuse for delay in applying existing knowledge as knowledge applied now will reap important dividends in the 21st century.

As far as screening is concerned, the impact of screening is likely to be prompt, but it is only likely to be important for cancers of the cervix and breast and possibly for oral cancer in some developing countries.

Finally it seems probable that the impact in improvements in therapy are immediate but likely to be small. In developing countries the impact of earlier diagnosis with effective local therapy could reduce deaths by as much as 20% to achieve survival rates approximately equivalent to those now seen in developed countries. However, resource lack may postpone this. In all countries pain relief for cancer is an important unmet need and is currently an important focus of the WHO cancer control program.

REFERENCES

1. Doll R, Peto R (1981). The causes of cancer: Quantitative estimates of avoidable risks of cancer in the United States today. J Natl Cancer Inst 66:1191-1308.
2. Miller AB (1984). The information explosion - the role of the epidemiologist. Cancer Forum 8:67-75.
3. Committee on Diet, Nutrition and Cancer (1982). Diet, nutrition and cancer. National Academy Press, Washington, D.C.
4. Risch H, Jain M, et al (1985). Dietary factors and the incidence of cancer of the stomach. Am J Epidemiol 122:947-959.
5. Jain M, Cook GM, et al (1980). A case-control study of diet and colo-rectal cancer. Int J Cancer 26:757-768.
6. Miller AB, Howe GR, et al (1983). Food items and food groups as risk factors in a case-control study of diet and colo-rectal cancer. Int J Cancer 32:155-161.
7. Graham S, Dayal H, et al (1978). Diet in the epidemiology of cancer of the colon and rectum. J Natl Cancer Inst 61:709-714.

8. Wattenberg LW (1981). Inhibitors of chemical carcino-
    gens. In: Burchenal JH, and Oettegen HF, eds. "Cancer:
    Achievements, Challenges, and prospects for the 1980's"
    Grune and Stratton, New York. Vol 1 pp 517-539.
9. Willett W, Stampfer MJ (1986). Total energy intake:
    Implications for epidemiologic analyses. Am J Epidemiol
    124:17-27.
10. Howe GR, Miller AB, et al (1986). Letter to the editor.
    Am J Epidemiol 124:157-159.
11. Newmark HL, Wargovich MJ et al (1984). Colon cancer
    and dietary fat, phosphate and calcium: A hypothesis.
    J Natl Cancer Inst 72:3513-3522.
12. Miller AB, Kelly A, et al (1978). A study of diet and
    breast cancer. Am J Epidemiol 107:499-509.
13. Howe GR (1985). The use of polytomous dual response
    data to increase power in case-control studies: An appli-
    cation to the association between dietary fat and breast
    cancer. J Chron Dis 38:663-670.
14. Lubin JH, Burns PE, et al (1981). Dietary factors and
    breast cancer risk. Int J Cancer 28:685-689.
15. Hislop TG, Goldman AJ, et al (1986). Childhood and
    recent eating patterns and risk of breast cancer. Cancer
    Detect Prev 9:47-58.
16. Lubin F, Ruder AM, et al (1985). Overweight and
    changes in weight throughout adult life in breast cancer
    etiology. Am J Epidemiol 122:579-588.
17. Kinlen L (1982). Meat and fat consumption and cancer
    mortality: A study of strict religious orders in Britain.
    Lancet 1:946-949.
18. Howe GR, Burch JD, et al (1980). Tobacco use, occupa-
    tion, coffee, various nutrients, and bladder cancer. J
    Natl Cancer Inst 64:701-713.
19. Winn DM, Blot WJ, et al (1981). Snuff dipping and oral
    cancer among women in the southern United States. New
    Engl J Med 305:745-749.
20. Miller AB (1985). Diet, nutrition and cancer. An
    epidemiological overview. J Nutr Growth and Cancer 2:159-
    171.
21. Gray N, Daube M, Eds. (1980). Guidelines for smoking
    control. 2nd edition. UICC Technical Report Series
    Vol. 52 International Union Against Cancer, Geneva, 1980.
22. Prorok PC, Chamberlain J, et al (1984). UICC workshop
    on the evaluation of screening programs for cancer. Int
    J Cancer 34:1-4.

23. Task Force (1976). Cervical cancer screening programs, The Walton report. Can Med Asso J 114:1003-1033.
24. Task Force (1982). Cervical cancer screening programs: summary of the 1982 Canadian task force report. Can Med Asso J 127:581-589.
25. Hakama M, Chamberlain J, et al (1985). Evaluation of screening programs for gynecological cancer. Br J Cancer 52:669-673.
26. Day NE, Moss S, et al (1986). Screening for squamous cervical cancer - the duration of low risk following negative cervical cytology and its implication for screening policies. (in preparation)
27. WHO Working Group (1986). Control of cancer of the cervix uteri. Bulletin Wor Hlth Org 64:607-618.
28. Miller AB, Howe GR, et al (1981). The national study of breast cancer screening. Protocol for a Canadian randomized controlled trial of screening for breast cancer in women. Clin Invest Med 4:277-358.
29. Miller AB, Bulbrook RD (1982). Screening, detection and diagnosis of breast cancer. Lancet 1:1109-1111.
30. Hall FM (1986). Screening mammography - potential problems on the horizon. New Eng J Med 314:53-55.
31. Chamberlain J, Day NE, et al (1986). UICC workshop on the project on evaluation of screening programs for gastrointestinal cancer. Int J Cancer 37:329-334.

RESEARCH ON SELECTED POPULATIONS

Advances in Cancer Control: The War on Cancer—
15 Years of Progress, pages 27–37
© 1987 Alan R. Liss, Inc.

A COMMUNITY-WIDE BREAST SELF-EXAM EDUCATION PROGRAM

John K. Worden, Brian S. Flynn, Laura J.
Solomon, Michael C. Costanza, Roger S. Foster
Jr., Anne L. Dorwaldt, Marilyn A. Driscoll,
Taka Ashikaga

Office of Health Promotion Research (J.K.W.,
B.S.F., A.L.D), and Departments of
Psychology (L.J.S), Biostatistics (M.C.C.,
T.A), Surgery and the Vermont Regional Cancer
Center (R.S.F.Jr., M.A.D), University of
Vermont, Burlington, Vermont 05405

Breast-self examination (BSE) is a method of
screening for breast cancer that every woman can
perform at home on a regular basis, at no cost.
Recent evidence shows that women who practice some
form of BSE and who are diagnosed as having breast
cancer have their cancers detected at an earlier
stage and have improved prospects for survival
compared with women who have not practiced BSE
(Foster and Costanza, 1984).

Programs to teach BSE have been implemented and
evaluated in a variety of settings but only rarely
on a community-wide basis. The few community-wide
studies have yielded promising results but were
conducted outside of North America and were not
rigorously evaluated (Aitken-Swan and Paterson,
1959; Gastrin, 1981). Although it has been
estimated that about 40% of the adult female
population performs some form of monthly BSE
(Worden et al, 1983; Sheley, 1983), recent studies
question whether the quality of BSE performed by
most women is adequate (Celentano and Holtzman,
1983; Sheley, 1983). To improve BSE quality,
palpation training techniques have been refined
(Baines, 1984), and methods to simplify BSE
training have been developed to facilitate adoption
of BSE as a regular health practice (Howe, 1981;
Mahoney and Csima, 1982). Several researchers have
identified important barriers to regular BSE
practice including anxiety about breast cancer,
lack of confidence in ability to perform BSE, and
difficulty remembering to do the behavior (Gallup,
1974; Stillman, 1977). Each must be considered
when planning a BSE training program.

The study reported in this paper has incorporated many of these recent developments in BSE education. A community-wide BSE training program was created. This program employed a simplified method of teaching BSE that emphasized breast palpation and addressed barriers to BSE practice. This study also included a community-wide assessment of the BSE training program so that changes in BSE practice could be measured for all women in a geographically-defined area, not just for women who received training voluntarily. Additionally, this study provides an opportunity to observe the effects of a BSE training program in a supportive community context, as a variety of community outreach techniques, including mass media, were implemented along with BSE training presentations.

The BSE training program developed in this study was based on an educational model proposed by Green and others (1980) and sought to increase both the frequency and quality of BSE among women in the community by attaining the following intermediate objectives: (1) improve BSE palpation skills; (2) enhance beliefs in the value of BSE, and in the woman's confidence that she can perform the behavior competently; and (3) increase social support (from family and friends) for conducting monthly BSE.

This paper reports on the initial results after one year of the BSE training program and does not encompass all aspects of the study. We report here on the exposure of women in the study communities to various parts of the educational program, improvements in BSE palpation skills, and changes in frequency and quality of BSE which have occurred after the first year of intervention.

BSE PROGRAM

The BSE training program consisted primarily of presentations by local home health agency nurses to small groups of women in clubs and organizations, worksites, churches, and gatherings of neighbors, friends, and relatives in women's homes. These

presentations were about an hour in length and
included: (1) a short dramatic film to trigger
discussion; (2) a brief discussion about breast
cancer, overcoming barriers to BSE, and the role of
BSE in early detection; (3) a five-minute
videotape demonstrating a simplified BSE technique;
(4) guided practice of breast palpation by
participants using silicone breast models; (5) a
question-and-answer period; and (6) distribution
of reminder materials, including a calendar
booklet, to enhance maintenance of monthly BSE. A
half-hour version of the program was designed for
worksites, clinics, and other contexts in which
time was limited.

The simplified BSE technique taught in this
program highlighted palpation while in a supine
position. Although palpation in the shower and
visual inspection of the breasts before a mirror
were mentioned, they were presented as supplements
to supine BSE. This concentration on palpation in
a single position enabled us to place strong
emphasis on the following specific palpation
techniques: using the flats of fingers, pressing
firmly, and covering of all the breast tissue and
the armpit area. These key points were presented
in the instructional videotape and reinforced
repeatedly by the nurses as women practiced on the
silicone breast models.

In addition to presentations to groups of
women, mass media were used to publicize the BSE
training sessions and to modify community norms in
support of learning BSE. Radio announcements
introduced the home health agency nurses as BSE
Program Leaders and presented testimonials by women
in the community who had attended training sessions
and could recommend them to other women. Newspaper
advertisements acknowledged women who had helped to
arrange BSE training sessions and publicized
upcoming presentations. Feature articles addressed
how BSE had benefited specific women in the
community. Television served two functions: (1) a
60-second spot depicted brief views of a training
session to enhance recruitment; and (2) a
half-hour program aired on a weekday evening near
the end of the intervention showed a complete
training session from which a woman could learn how

to do BSE in the convenience and privacy of her home.

One of the critical aspects of this program was the recruitment of women into BSE training presentations. Using a recruitment plan developed and successfully utilized in a Vermont BSE education study in the mid-1970s (Worden *et al*, 1983), the BSE Program Leaders attempted to reach many women in the community through women's groups and organizations. However, with many women working outside the home in the mid-1980s, fewer women appeared to belong to organized community groups. Worksite recruitment proved limited because many women in small Vermont communities work in settings having few employees, and because the private nature of the behavior made training in these worksites less appealing. To stimulate greater participation, we established support groups of enthusiastic local women who had attended our BSE training sessions and were willing to volunteer for a three-month period to help with recruitment. The most important contribution of these women to the program was organization of numerous training presentations in their homes, which boosted recruitment figures substantially.

STUDY DESIGN AND ASSESSMENT

The research design of this two-year study is shown in Figure 1. Six communities in Vermont, ranging in population from 4,000 to 8,000, were selected as target populations from a state-wide list of communities through a systematic procedure which considered numbers of adult women, educational attainment, religious affiliations, and geographic dispersion. All six communties received a baseline survey (Flynn *et al*, 1986), and the four communities with the most similar levels of BSE frequency were retained for the study. The four participating communities were randomly assigned to each of the following conditions shown in Figure 1: Experimental 1 (E1), receiving BSE training in the first year followed by BSE maintenance in the second year and annual surveys; Experimental 2 (E2), receiving BSE training in the first year and annual surveys but no new program in the second year; Control 1 (C1), receiving no programs but receiving annual surveys; and Control 2 (C2), receiving only pretest and posttest surveys as a low-measurement control. This paper reports initial follow-up results of the Fall 1985 survey and therefore does not address the BSE maintenance program nor does it include data from C2.

Community	Summer 1985		Fall 1985		Fall 1986
E1	TS*	BSE Training	TS, HS*	Maintenance	TS, HS
E2	TS	BSE Training	TS, HS		TS, HS
C1	TS		TS, HS		TS, HS
C2	TS				TS, HS

* TS: Telephone Survey; HS: Home Survey

Figure 1. Study Design

The surveys indicated in Figure 1 are of two types. The first was a telephone survey of a representative sample of at least 325 women aged 20 and older from each community, selected by random digit dialing. The telephone survey measured BSE frequency and quality, beliefs about breast cancer and BSE, previous experience with breast cancer and breast cancer screening, and exposure to BSE education, including mass media messages. The second survey was a brief home interview of a 50% sub-sample of the telephone sample to measure BSE palpation skills, using a poster-board drawing of a woman's chest to assess coverage and silicone breast models to measure palpation technique. For the pretest in Summer 1984, only the telephone survey was conducted; a total of 1064 women were interviewed in the E1, E2, and C1 communities. In the Fall 1985 survey, 1018 women were called who agreed at the end of the first survey to be interviewed again. Of these women 11.6% could not be reached again, and 9.2% refused to be interviewed, leaving a sample of 806 women. Home interviews were conducted with 454 women who had indicated in the follow-up telephone survey that they had ever done BSE; 36.4% of those asked to participate in the home survey on the telephone refused to be visited at home, and 4.9% refused when the interviewer arrived at the home. These percentages were higher than expected. Refusals appeared to be related to the presence of the BSE program, with 31.9% and 32.3% refusing in E1 and E2 communities and 46.0% refusing in the C1 community. This pattern tends to reduce the likelihood of finding hypothesized differences in response measures among study communities, with a more select group of women consenting to participate in the control area than in the experimental areas.

ONE-YEAR RESULTS

Responses to the follow-up telephone survey indicated that women living in the E1 and E2 communities recalled exposure to much higher levels of BSE education and information than did women in the C1 community. Among women in the E1 and E2 communities, 41% and 39%, respectively, recalled attending a BSE training presentation, with no women in the C1 community recalling such participation. Approximately 45% of the women in the E1 and E2 communities recalled seeing something in the newspaper about BSE that was generated by our program, and 23% recalled seeing something on television about BSE from our program. There was a difference regarding radio, with 48% of the women in the E1 community (having a strong local station) and 26% of the women in the E2 community (having a more distant regional station) recalling something about BSE that was generated by our program. In comparison, only 3% of the women in the C1 community recall hearing or seeing something about BSE from our program on one or more mass media. Recall of BSE education and information from sources outside of our program was generally the same across all three study communities.

BSE Palpation Skills

The home interview involved direct observation of each woman's proficiency in performing breast palpation on the poster-board drawing of a woman's chest (to assess coverage) and on silicone breast models with five simulated lumps embedded in them (to assess finger technique). Table 1 indicates the proportion of women in the C1 and experimental communities who performed each skill adequately. A significantly larger proportion of women (p<.05) in the experimental communities performed these skills adequately compared to the C1 community, except for making small finger movements (p<.10).

Table 1: BSE palpation skills performed adequately by women in C1 and experimental communities and by non-participants and participants in group BSE training (%).

BSE Palpation Skills	C1	E	Non-Participants	Participants
Using flats of fingers	35	57	46	70
Pressing firmly	45	56	37	75
Making small finger movements	47 *	56 *	43	69
Using a consistent pattern	63	74	62	86
Covering entire breast	20	56	44	69

* p<.10; all other comparisons p<.05 using chi-square test.

To help assess the importance of participation in the BSE training program, Table 1 also indicates the proportion of women (living in the experimental communities) and not participating in the programs who performed each skill adequately, and the proportion of those women participating in the programs who performed each skill adequately. There was a significantly higher level of proficiency for women who had participated in the program compared to those who had not participated (all p<.05).

As a second measure of BSE palpation skills, we counted the number of lumps that women correctly detected of the five placed in various parts of each silicone model. Women were asked to palpate two models; therefore, they had a possible maximum score of ten lumps detected. As indicated in Figure 2, women in the C1 community discovered a mean of 2.85 lumps and women in the experimental communities discovered a mean of 3.66 lumps, significantly more (p<.01 based on analysis of variance) than the C1 community. The mean number of lumps palpated by women who had or had not participated in the women's group BSE training program is also shown in Figure 2. While, non-participants discovered a mean of 2.78 lumps, participants discovered a mean of 4.61 lumps. This difference was significant (p<.0001).

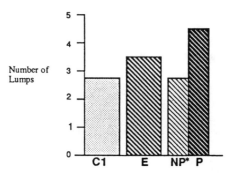

Figure 2: Number of lumps discovered
in silicone breast models by women in
C1 and experimental communities
and among non-participants and
participants in experimental
communities.

* NP: Non-participants; P: Participants

BSE Frequency and Quality

The BSE frequency data were dichotomized into
monthly (four or more times in the last six months)
versus less than monthly. Changes in monthly BSE
performance from baseline to the Fall 1985
follow-up survey between the experimental (E1 and
E2) and control (C1) communities were studied using
loglinear models. These analyses indicated that
the model in which the treatment variable and
baseline BSE frequency were independent given the
follow-up BSE frequency provided an excellent fit
to the data (p>.90). This model permitted the
direct comparison of the follow-up BSE frequency
data between the experimental and control
communities. There was a significant difference in
favor of the experimental communities (p< .01).
Figure 3 shows that the proportion of respondents
reporting that they have practiced BSE monthly
increased from 48.0% to 58.0% in the experimental
communities compared to a slight corresponding
increase from 42.4% to 44.1% in the C1 community.

To determine BSE quality, we used a method similar to that of Celentano and Holtzman (1983) to construct a checklist of appropriate steps for conducting breast palpation while lying down. These checklist components included: putting hand behind head, using opposite hand, using flats of fingers, using a consistent pattern, including the armpit area, putting a prop under the shoulder, and pressing firmly. Figure 4 indicates the mean number of these steps that were mentioned by women in the experimental and C1 communities when asked to describe their BSE technique. In the experimental communities, the mean of appropriate steps increased in one year from 1.06 to 1.54. In the C1 community, the mean number of correct steps decreased from 1.17 to 1.04. The difference in change scores was statistically significant ($p<.05$, based on analysis of variance).

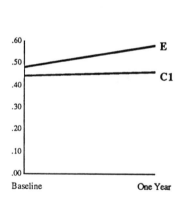

Figure 3. Proportion of women in experimental and C1 communities who were performing monthly BSE ($\geq$4 times in past 6 months) at baseline and one year after the start of the BSE education program.

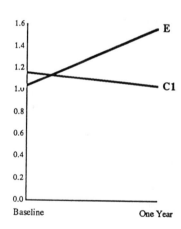

Figure 4. Number of BSE steps (performing palpation while lying down) reported by women in experimental and C1 communities at baseline and one year after the start of the BSE education program.

CONCLUSIONS

The primary BSE training approach in this study was through group instruction held in the context of a women's club or organization, a worksite, a

church, or a group gathering at a woman's home.
Recruitment of women to participate in the group
training was accomplished initially by home health
agency nurses in direct contact with club and
organization leaders and with employers; however,
a more successful approach also was undertaken
through the organization of women's support groups
whose members set up training sessions for women in
their own homes. With these recruitment
approaches, supported by a mass media campaign,
about 40% of the women living in the communities
offered the BSE training actually participated in
the group training program over a one-year period.

A simplified, one-step BSE was taught in the
group training program with an emphasis on guided
practice of specific, well-defined palpation
skills. The importance of skills practice is
reflected in results which showed that women who
actually attended the BSE training presentations
could perform palpation more completely and
discovered a significantly greater number of lumps
than did women who did not attend the training
presentations.

An important feature of the study design was the
ability to measure the community-wide effects of
BSE group training combined with mass media
support. We conclude that the program achieved a
community-wide improvement in BSE performance
because at the one-year assessment significantly
more women in the experimental communities than in
the control community practiced monthly BSE (i.e.,
performed BSE at least four times in the past six
months), indicated a higher quality of BSE, used
four out of the five palpation skills correctly,
and discovered more lumps in the silicone breast
model. While the immediate impact of this BSE
training program is apparent, this study also will
permit further analyses of the relative BSE
performance of women living in experimental and
control communities, and those who do and do not
participate in face-to-face training, in order to
provide a more complete picture of how women
respond to a community-wide BSE education program.

REFERENCES

Aitken-Swan J, Paterson R (1959). Assessment of the results of five years of cancer education. Brit Med J.1:708.

Baines CJ (1984). Breast self-examination: The doctor's role. Hosp Pract 19:120-127.

Celentano DD, Holtzman D (1983). Breast self-examination competency: An analysis of self-reported practice and associated characterisitcs. Am J Public Health 73:1321-1323.

Flynn BS, Costanza MC, Worden JK, Solomon LJ (1986). Diagnostic study for breast self-examination education program shows importance of confidence and social support. Paper presented at American Public Health Association Annual Meeting, Las Vegas, Nevada.

Foster RS Jr, Costanza MC (1984). Breast self-examination practices and breast cancer survival. Cancer 53:999-1005.

Gallup Organization (1974). Women's attitudes regarding breast cancer. Occup Health Nurs 22:20.

Gastrin G. (1981). Breast Cancer Control. Almqvist and Wiksell International, Stockhholm, Sweden.

Green LW, Kreuter MW, Deeds SG, Partridge KB (1980). Health Education - A Diagnostic Approach. Mayfield, Palo Alto, California.

Howe HL (1981). Enhancing the effectiveness of media messages promoting regular breast self-examination. Public Health Rep 96:134-142.

Mahoney L, Csima A (1982). Efficiency of palpation in clinical detection of breast cancer. CMA J 127:729-730.

Sheley JF (1983). Inadequate transfer of breast cancer self-detection technology. Am J Public Health 73:1318-1320.

Stillman MJ (1977). Women's health beliefs about breast cancer and breast self-examination. Nurs Res 26:121-127.

Worden JK, Costanza MC, Foster RS Jr, Lang SP, Tidd CA (1983). Content and context in health education: Persuading women to perform breast self-examination. Prev Med 12:331-339.

Advances in Cancer Control: The War on Cancer—
15 Years of Progress, pages 39–51
© 1987 Alan R. Liss, Inc.

TOWARD EFFECTIVE APPLICATION OF EFFICACIOUS
CANCER CONTROL INTERVENTIONS

Nicole Urban, Sc.D., Beti Thompson, Ph.D.,
Electra Pasket, M.P.H.

Fred Hutchinson Cancer Research Center,
Cancer Prevention Research Unit, 1124
Columbia Street, Seattle, Washington, 98103.

INTRODUCTION

The use of mammography in screening for breast cancer
has been shown to reduce breast cancer mortality between
30% (Shapiro et al, 1982) and 41% (Tabar et al, 1985) in
women over the age of 50. Accordingly, the American
Cancer Society recommends annual mammography for all
women aged 50 and above, as well as annual physical
examination of the breasts for all women aged 40 and
over.

However, fewer than 10% of family physicians
recommend an annual mammogram for asymptomatic women over
the age of 50 (Cummings et al, 1983). Physicians are
reluctant to refer women for annual mammography, in part
because of its high cost which is not generally covered
by health insurance. Although mammography has been shown
to be efficacious in several studies (Shapiro et al,
1971; Tabar et al, 1985; Colette et al, 1984; Verbeek et
al, 1984), its cost effectiveness has not been
demonstrated. In particular, the relative cost-
effectiveness of alternative screening strategies has not
been assessed, leaving insurers, organizations,
physicians and women uncertain how to proceed with
respect to screening for breast cancer.

METHODS

The best approach to evaluating the relative
cost-effectiveness of alternative screening strategies
is to conduct a series of randomized trials. In fact,
several such trials are now in progress (Miller et al.
1981; Roberts et al, 1984). However, it is not feasible
to conduct a randomized trial of every possible screening
strategy. Thus, it is useful to estimate, based on
current knowledge and simple modeling techniques, the
marginal cost and marginal health benefit of variations
in those screening strategies which have been tested for
efficacy. Such a model is under development at the
Cancer Control Research Unit in Seattle (Urban et al,
1985).

The purpose of the model is to find ways to improve
the cost-effectiveness relative to the outcome-
effectiveness of interventions assumed to be efficacious
in reducing mortality from breast cancer. Combinations
of mammography, physical examination of the breasts, and
instruction in breast self-examination (BSE) at various
time intervals are compared in terms of their impact on
mortality in a defined population and their detection
costs per woman at risk and per death averted. Savings
in treatment costs attributable to earlier detection of
breast cancer are not taken into account in this
preliminary version of the model. Ten alternative
screening strategies, in addition to a baseline, are
compared (Figure 1).

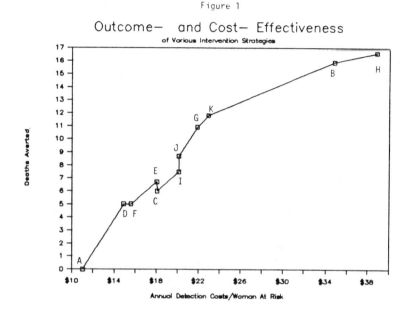

Figure 1

Outcome— and Cost— Effectiveness
of Various Intervention Strategies

Each box in Figure 1 represents a screening strategy. It can be seen from Figure 1 that the relationship between mortality reduction and detection costs exhibits diminishing marginal returns: increases in expenditures on breast cancer detection result in less than proportional increases in deaths averted, for strategies that are efficient in the sense that they avert as many deaths as possible for a given expenditure. The model suggests that strategies F, C and I should not be employed because they are inefficient. For the same annual expenditures per woman at risk, more deaths can be averted by strategies E and J than by strategies C and I respectively. Similarly, strategy F should not be chosen because strategy D averts as many deaths at lower costs. Comparison between strategies J and E is less straightforward, however, since strategy J averts more

deaths at greater cost. To choose between strategies J
and E it is necessary to decide how much society is
willing to pay to avert another breast cancer death. It
is clear from Figure 1 that among efficient strategies,
there is a tradeoff between outcome-effectiveness and
cost-effectiveness: Strategies B and H are the most
outcome-effective but the least cost-effective.

The usual approach to improving outcome-effectiveness
is to combine several detection modalities, keeping the
interval between screens short and including the entire
target population. This is the strategy that was adopted
by the Health Insurance Plan (HIP) of Greater New York
(Shapiro et al, 1971) and by the Breast Cancer Detection
Demonstration Project (BCDDP) (Baker 1982). One means of
improving cost-effectiveness is to use a single modality
(e.g. mammography alone) and a longer screening interval
for mammography. This is the strategy adopted in Sweden
where women over the age of 50 are screened by
single-view mammography alone at an average interval of
33 months (Tabar et al, 1985). A second means of
improving cost-effectiveness is to exclude from the
screening program women at relatively low risk of breast
cancer, or to screen such women at longer intervals.
This is the strategy in use at Group Health Cooperative
(GHC) of Puget Sound, where the highest-risk women
are receiving mammography annually and the lowest-risk
women are not receiving mammography at all, while medium-
and low-risk women are receiving mammography at three and
five year intervals respectively (Carter et al, 1983).

A third means of improving cost-effectiveness, not
currently in use to our knowledge, is to stagger the
application of different detection modalities in order to
avoid redundancy. Since mammography can be expected to
detect close to 90% of cancers detectable by either
mammography or physical examination, the use of physical
examination in synchronous combination with mammography
yields little additional benefit. However, use of

physical examination in years two and four when mammography is used biannually in years one and three is useful, since physical examination can be expected to detect approximately 56% of the cancers that would be detectable by either mammography or physical examination. Estimates of redundancy in screening modalities are based on data from the BCDDP shown in Table 1 (Baker, 1982).

Table 1

RELATIVE CONTRIBUTION OF MAMMOGRAPHY, PHYSICAL EXAMINATION, AND SELF-DETECTION IN A SCREENING PROGRAM

	Number	Percent of All Cases	Percent of Cases Detected at Screening
Mammography Only	1481	34.4	41.6
Mammography and Physical Examination	1683	39.1	47.3
Physical Examination Only	308	7.2	8.7
Unknown (screening)	85	2.0	2.4
Interval cases (within one year of last screen)	744	17.3	
	4301	100%	100%

Our approach to modeling the effectiveness and costs of alternative screening strategies requires assumptions about 1) the incidence of breast cancer; 2) the relative risk of breast cancer in subgroups of the target population; 3) the probability of detection in each stage, as a function of the mode of detection and the time since last negative screen by each mode of detection; 4) the probability of exposure to each screening modality in the current period; 5) the probability of exposure to various services and incurrance of their resulting costs as a function of exposure to screening modalities, 6) the costs of detection and related services, and 7) the relationship between breast cancer mortality and the distribution by stage of incident cancers.

Although simpler, the approach is based conceptually on the work of David Eddy (Eddy, 1980). Still in development, the model depends for its input on parameters which can be estimated in the context of a non-experimental breast cancer screening program. Results reported here should be viewed as preliminary, since they are based on estimates taken from the literature. For example, estimates employed of the probability of detection in stage one (without ancillary node involvement) as a function of mode of detection and time since last mammogram, based on data reported in the literature (Hugueley and Brown, 1981 and Shapiro et al, 1971), are given in Table 2. Assumptions about the costs of various detection and related services are given in Table 3.

Table 2

PROBABILITY OF EARLY DETECTION AS A FUNCTION OF MODE OF DETECTION AND TIME SINCE LAST MAMMOGRAM HOLDING CONSTANT TIME SINCE LAST PE AND BSE INSTRUCTION

Time Since Last Mammogram	Asymptomatic			Symptomatic
	Mammogram	Physical Exam	BSE	
12 months	.883	.611	.657	.570
24 months				
36 months				
60+ months	.781	.541	.581	.504

Table 3

Unit Costs of Detection and Related Services
Employed in Breast Cancer Screening Model

SERVICE	UNIT COST
BSE Minimal Instruction	$ 1
BSE Interactive Instruction	5
Screening Mammogram	30
Diagnostic Mammogram	100
Screening Physical Exam	5
Physical Exam for Symptoms	35
Consult for Suspicious Mammogram	50
Biopsy with Surgical Consultation	500

RESULTS

The ten screening strategies are compared in groups
of three. The first group represents applications of
single detection modalities annually. The three are
shown in Figure 2. Strategy B represents annual
mammography for all women. Strategy C represents annual
BSE instruction for all women. Strategy D represents
annual physical examination for all women. It is assumed
that 75% of women receiving BSE instruction in the
current period actually perform BSE for a year and that
24% of the remaining women perform BSE as a result of
previous instruction in BSE. Strategy A represents a
baseline situation, in which 24% of women perform BSE,
3% receive mammography, and 31% receive physical
examination of the breasts in the current year. It is
also assumed that 90% of women participate in the
programs represented by strategies B, C, and D, the rest
exhibiting baseline behavior.

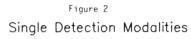

Figure 2
Single Detection Modalities

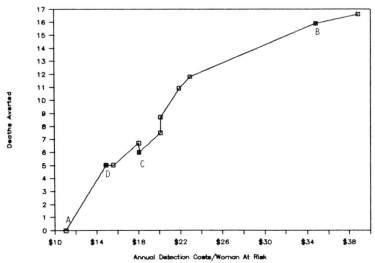

As can be seen from Figure 2, annual mammography (strategy B) is highly outcome-effective: it averts 15.9 deaths per year in a hypothetical population of 100,000 women age 50 and above at a cost of about 3.5 million dollars. The marginal cost per death averted of this strategy, relative to baseline, is approximately $150,000.

Annual physical examination of the breasts (strategy D) is highly cost-effective: it averts five deaths at a cost of just under 1.5 million dollars, or a marginal cost of $77,000 per death averted relative to baseline. It should be noted that even in the absence of a systematic breast cancer program, detection of breast cancer costs approximately $11 per woman at risk, due to baseline utilization rates. Annual BSE instruction (strategy C) is not considered because it is inefficient relative to strategy E, as shown in Figure 1. A relevant question is, what is the relative cost-effectiveness of annual mammography relative to annual physical examination? It averts 10.9 additional deaths for about 2 million additional dollars for a marginal cost per death averted (relative to annual physical examination

rather than to baseline) of about $183,000. Annual
mammography should be employed rather than annual
physical examination if society is willing to pay
$183,000 to avert a breast cancer death.

The second group of strategies considered includes
three strategies involving mammography alone employed at
various intervals, shown in Figure 3. Strategy E
represents mammography employed at a three-year interval
for all women. This strategy averts 6.7 deaths for
approximately 1.8 million dollars in a hypothetical
population of 100,000 women age 50 and over, for a
marginal cost per death averted (relative to baseline) of
$105,000. Strategy F represents mammography applied at a
sixteen-month interval for women with a relative risk of
breast cancer of 3.0 (high-risk women) and a three-year
interval for women with a relative risk of 2.0
(medium-risk women), with no screening for women with
baseline risk (low risk). This strategy is not considered
because it is inefficient relative to annual physical
examination for all women (strategy D; see Figure 2).

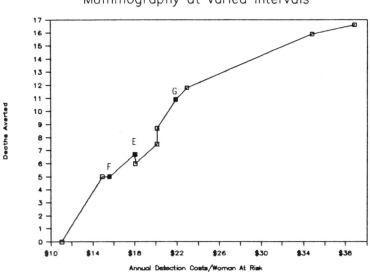

Figure 3
Mammography at Varied Intervals

Strategy G represents annual mammography for
high-risk women, mammography at a 16-month interval for
medium-risk women, and mammography at a three-year

interval for low-risk women. This strategy averts 10.9
deaths and costs about 2.2 million dollars in a
hypothetical population of 100,000 women aged 50 and
over. Relative to baseline, it averts 10.9 deaths for a
marginal cost of $99,000 per death averted. Relative to
mammography at a three-year interval for all women, it
averts 4.2 deaths for a marginal cost per death averted
of $92,000. Since there are no diminishing returns
between strategies E and G, strategy G is preferred to
strategy E. That is, outcome and cost-effectiveness are
both better for strategy G than for strategy E.

The third and last group of screening strategies
considered includes four strategies in which screening
modalities are combined at varied intervals with and
without staggering in their application, shown in Figure
4. Strategy H represents mammography, BSE instruction,
and physical examination in combination annually for all
women. This strategy averts 16.6 deaths and costs about
3.9 million dollars in a hypothetical population of women
aged 50 and over. Relative to annual mammography alone
for all women (strategy B, Figure 2) it averts only .7
additional death for about $400,000, or $572,000 per
additional death averted. Thus its cost-effectiveness is
low, due to diminishing returns to efforts to detect
breast cancers.

Figure 4

Combinations of Screening Modalities

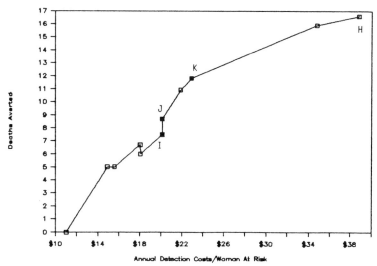

Strategy I represents mammography, physical examination, and BSE instruction in synchronous combination at three-year intervals. This strategy is not considered because it is inefficient relative to strategy J, which represents the same three modalities applied at staggered three-year intervals. The latter strategy averts 8.7 deaths for a total cost of 2 million dollars in our hypothetical population of 100,000. Relative to baseline, it averts 8.7 deaths for a marginal cost per death averted of $105,000. Since a varied interval for mammography alone (strategy G, Figure 3) averts 10.9 deaths for a marginal cost of $99,000 per death averted relative to baseline, strategy G is preferred to Strategy J (staggering of three modalities) for its greater outcome- and cost-effectiveness.

Strategy K, the last strategy considered, combines the strengths of strategies J and G in order to improve outcome-effectiveness while maintaining cost-effectiveness. As in strategy G, high- and medium-risk women are screened annually and at a sixteen-month interval respectively. However, the low-risk women receive staggered mammography, physical examination, and BSE instruction at three-year intervals as in strategy J.

It can be seen from Figure 4 that strategy K averts 11.8 deaths annually for a total cost of 2.3 million dollars, improving outcome-effectiveness (relative to strategy G) by averting 0.9 more deaths at a marginal cost per additional death averted of $118,000. Thus strategy K is preferred to other strategies clustering in the lower left quadrant of Figure 1 if society is willing to pay $118,000 to avert a breast cancer death. Similarly, the choice between annual mammagraphy for all women (strategy B) and the combined approach represented by strategy K depends upon how much society is willing to pay to avert breast cancer deaths. The former averts 4.1 additional deaths, at a marginal cost of $289,000 per additional death averted, relative to the latter.

DISCUSSION

In general, society should expect to pay more at the margin for preventive programs that save additional lives. Choosing a strategy that is cost-effective involves first, eliminating from consideration strategies that are inefficient, and second, considering mortality reductions in relation to their marginal costs. Society must decide how much it is worth to avert another breast cancer death, when those that can be averted relatively inexpensively have already been averted.

The analysis offered above should be viewed as preliminary in several ways. First, it is based on estimates from the literature, some of which are outdated; mammography has improved dramatically since the 1960's (Baker, 1982). Second, the model is still under development and does not yet take into consideration savings in treatment costs which may be attributable to earlier detection of breast cancer. Third, cost-effectiveness of alternative preventive strategies is best evaluated in terms of marginal cost per quality-adjusted year of life saved (Russell, 1986). The model does not yet yield these calculations.

Nevertheless, the authors believe that the conceptual framework described and the preliminary analyses performed suggest some options for breast cancer screening that may warrant further consideration.

REFERENCES

Baker LH (1982). Breast Cancer Detection Demonstration Project; Five year summary report. Ca-A Can J for Clinicians 32 (4):194-225.
Carter AP, Thompson RS, Bourdeau R, Ferguson G, Mustin H, Straley H, Andenes J (1983). Report on Early Detection of Breast Cancer; Implications for Group Health Cooperative of Puget Sound.

Colette HJA, Day NE, Rombach JJ, de Waard F (1984). Evaluation of screening for breast cancer in a non-randomized study (the DOM project) by means of a case-control study. Lancet i:1224-26.

Cummings KM, Funch DP, Mettlin C, Jennings E (1983). Family physicians' beliefs about breast cancer screening by mammography. J Fam Prac 17(6):1029-1034.

Eddy DM (1980). "Screening for Cancer: Theory, Analysis, and Design" New Jersey, Englewood Clitts: Prentice-Hall, Inc.

Miller AB, Howe GR, Wall C (1981). The national study of breast cancer screening. Clinical and Investigative Medicine 4 (3/4):227-258.

Roberts MM, Alexander FE, Anderson TJ, et al (1984). The Edinburgh randomized trial of screening for breast cancer: Description of method. Br J Can 50:1-6.

Russell LB (1986). "Is Prevention Better than Cure?" Washington DC: The Brookings Institute.

Shapiro S, Strax P, Venet L (1971). Periodic breast cancer screening in reducing mortality from breast cancer. JAMA 215(11):1777-1785.

Shapiro S, Venet W, Strax P, et al (1982). Ten- to fourteen-year effect of screening on breast cancer mortality. JNCI 69(2):349-355.

Tabar L, Gad A, Holmberg LH, Ljungquist U, Fagerberg CJG, Baldetorp L, Grontoft O, Lundstrom B, Manson JC (1985). Reduction in mortality from breast cancer after mass screening with mammography. Lancet 8433:829-832.

Urban N, Avlon E, Thompson B (1985). "The Use of Health Statistics in Predicting the Effects of Intervention Programs to Increase Early Detection of Breast Cancer", proceedings of the Public Health Conference on Records and Statistics, DHHS Pub. No. (PHS) 86-1214.

Verbeek ALM, Holland R, Sturmans F, Mravunac M, Sturmans F, Day NE (1984). Reduction of breast cancer mortality through mass screening with modern mammography. The Lancet:1222-1226.

Advances in Cancer Control: The War on Cancer—
15 Years of Progress, pages 53–65
© 1987 Alan R. Liss, Inc.

ISSUES IMPACTING ON ACCEPTANCE AND COMPLIANCE IN A
COMMUNITY BASED COLORECTAL SCREENING PROGRAM

Diane Gordon, R. N., MPH and Gordon L. Doty, M.D.,
Providence Medical Center, Portland, Oregon 97213

INTRODUCTION

Colorectal cancers are the second most common cancers
in both sexes and the second leading cause of death due
to cancer in the United States today, second only to lung
cancer. According to the American Cancer Society
estimates, in 1986 140,000 new cases of colorectal cancer
will be diagnosed and 60,000 colorectal cancer deaths
will occur (1986 ACS Cancer Facts and Figures).

The prevalence of colorectal cancer in men and women at
average risk in the general population over age 40 is 1-2
per 1000. (Schottenfield & Winawer 1982). There has not
been any significant change in mortality from this
disease over the last fifty years with an overall five
year survival rate of around 44%. The five year survival
rate climbs to approximately 75% when colorectal cancer
is discovered and treated in an early stage, usually when
patients are asymptomatic. (Sherlock & Winawer, 1984).

COLORECTAL HEALTH CHECK PROGRAM

In 1984, the American Cancer Society instituted a
national three year Colorectal Health Check Program
(CHEC) to increase public awareness of colorectal cancer
and to educate lay and professional groups about the
disease. The American Cancer Society recommends three
screening tests for the early detection of colorectal
cancer in asymptomatic individuals over age 40-50. These

include annual digital rectal examinations beginning at age 40 years; annual fecal guaiac screening beginning at age 50 years; and two sigmoidoscopies one year apart starting at age fifty, and if these are negative, then subsequent sigmoidoscopies every three to five years (Sherlock and Winawer, 1984).

It has been suggested that when a colorectal screening program is introduced into a community, major educational benefits occur including interest in and discussions regarding lifestyle, diet and the overall public health importance of colorectal cancer, and that there is increased awareness of the important early warning signs that would require medical attention (Winawer, 1985).

METHODOLOGY

In April of 1985 and again in August, Providence Cancer Center and the Oregon Division of the American Cancer Society, Inc., offered a free blood stool screening to the public as part of the overall Colorectal Health Check Program.

The main goal and focus of the April screening program was to provide education both to the public and health professionals especially concerning the need for early detection. This was accomplished through a community-wide program publicized via radio, community flyers and articles in community and senior newspapers. Partici-pants were required to come into the hospital to receive their blood stool testing kits. Programs were also held in the community at various senior centers. Individual-ized instruction and education was provided, for the most part, by retired volunteer nurses. A slide presentation prepared by the ACS was also utilized in group presenta-tions. Physician participation was invited through a pre-established referral mechanism.

The program was repeated again in August, 1985, as a result of anticipated interest in the diagnosis of colon cancer in President Reagan. The focus of the educational approach was not individualized, as in the first screen-ing and the majority of participants received their home testing kits and educational materials through a direct mailing after an initial telephone screen to determine basic eligibility and take requests for kits.

Screening eligibility was determined following the ACS guidelines. All persons over age 40 were offered the free blood stool testing. Those persons with any symptoms of rectal bleeding, hemorrhoids, personal history of cancer, ulcerative colitis or familial polyposis were discouraged from taking the test and referred to their family physician for follow-up. Dietary instructions were printed on each testing kit and were also reviewed with each person receiving the home tests.

All kits were distributed with return mail envelopes to be sent back to the Providence Medical Center laboratory for processing. Participants were notified by mail of test results. All participants were required to complete a release form (consent to participate) which included a name of a physician to whom positive results could be sent. Follow-up forms were sent on all positive screens to the referring physician. Information collected included demographics on the participants, diagnostic work-up, stage of disease if detected, and treatment information. This data was analyzed to examine the impact of the overall screening program and also to provide information to the American College of Surgeons national Patient Care Evaluation Study being conducted in cooperation with the ACS CHEC Program.

The screening program was also offered to all hospital employees and volunteers meeting the eligibility criteria.

RESULTS

Twelve hundred guaiac testing kits were distributed free of charge in the April screen and 3500 were distributed again in August for a total of 4700 kits. In the first screen 520 or 43% were returned; in the second screen 1165 or 33% were returned (Table 1). Compliance for the total screen was 1685 responses or 36%.

TABLE 1. Colorectal Screening Participation

	April,1985	August,1985	Total
No. kits distributed	1200	3500	4700
No. responses	520	1165	1685
% responses	43%	33%	36%

A total of 92 screens were positive (5.5%). The average age of the patients with positive screens was 64; forty-nine (53%) were women and forty-three (47%) were male. Diagnostic workup was done on 80 of these patients. Ten persons refused further workup in spite of multiple efforts to convince them to do so. Two patients received no further workup due to other medical conditions. Follow up information was received from physicians on all but two of the patients seen.

Fifty-two of the positive patients were asymptomatic at the time of follow-up and nine presented with symptoms.- Physician work-up was variable. Eighteen patients had repeat blood stool tests alone; only 15 patients received a colonoscopy as part of their work up, the cancer patients had a more comprehensive work up.

TABLE 2. Physician Work-up of Patients with Positive Screens

Repeat Stool Blood Only		18
Repeat Stool Blood + Anoscope		1
Repeat Stool Blood + Rectal Exam		3
Repeat Stool Blood + BE		2
Repeat Stool Blood + BE & UGI		1
Barium Enema Only		1
Sigmoidoscopy 25 cm.	10	(1 cancer)
Sigmoidoscopy + BE	7	
Sigmoidoscopy + BE + UGI	6	
Sigmoidoscopy 60 cm.	8	
Sigmoidoscopy + BE	4	(1 cancer)
Sigmoidoscopy + BE + UGI	2	
Colonoscopy	11	(1 cancer)
Colonoscopy + BE	2	(1 cancer)
Colonoscopy + UGI	2	

In 44 positive patients, no abnormalities could be found; 30 had abnormalities other than cancer including 6 with polyps. One colon cancer (stage one) and three rectal cancers (stage 0 insitu in a polyp, stage one and stage three) were found.

TABLE 3. Colorectal Screening Results

Patients with positive Coloscreen	92
No Abnormalities found	44
"Benign" lesions	30
Not evaluated	14
Cancers detected	4

TABLE 4. Identifiable Abnormalities

Cancer		4	
Colon	(1)		(Stage I)
Rectum	(3)		
			(Stage 0)
			(Stage I)
			(Stage III)
Benign Lesions		30	
Hemorrhoids		10	
Diverticula		9	
Polyps		6	
Hiatal Hernia		2	
Duodenal Ulcer			
Healed		2	
Duodenal Ulcer			
Active		1	
Duodenitis		1	

In patients with cancer the number of positive slides increased with more advanced disease.

TABLE 5. Positive Slides, Cancer Patients

1 / 9	Stage 0
3 / 9	Stage I
4 / 9	Stage I
9 / 9	Stage III

DISCUSSION

Almost all published screening trials have been uncontrolled. (Simon, 1985) in a review of such trials found an overall detection of about 3-20 colorectal malignancies for every 10,000 people enrolled, with only 5-10% of occult blood reactions being due to cancer. Our screening program showed similar results; with 9 cancers per 10,000 persons enrolled and a predictive value for the test of 4%.

As with other uncontrolled screening trials there is a wide variation in compliance rates, ranging from 15-98% (Simon, 1985) with data from some mass screening programs showing compliance to be less than 30% (Winawer, et al, 1983). Our first screening program which utilized individualized instruction and education had a compliance rate of 43%; our second screening program - utilizing mailed instruction and education - had a compliance rate of 33% (p< .01).* This was statistically significant.

Multiple factors appear to affect how successfully a target population cooperates with a cancer detection program. Complex sociodemographic factors, individual health beliefs and motivations all are involved. Perceived personal susceptibility to the disease as well as perceived benefit from a screening program on an individual basis are known to influence a person's decision to participate in a screening program. (Macrae, 1984; Halper, et al, 1980). Silman and Mitchell (1984) found that the major reason for non-participation in colorectal screening programs was lack of a perceived individual need for screening in asymptomatic persons although there was an appreciation for the potential of an overall community health benefit. They concluded that there was a need for individualized health education in such screening programs. Other authors have recommended the same (Messner, et al, 1986; Silman and Mitchell, 1984).

A study conducted by the ACS on public attitudes of persons towards colon and rectal cancer revealed disturbing perceptions regarding the disease and participation in detection and treatment programs (ACS 1983). One significant finding was the perception that most people

* Blacock Herbert M Jr., <u>Social Statistics,</u> 2nd Ed., 1972.

did not consider tests for detection of colon and rectal cancer to be part of a physical examination.

This emphasizes the need for physicians to make these tests part of their physical exams and educate their patients to the importance such screening exams. Other findings in the survey showed that people do not view colorectal cancer as important; women regard it as a male disease and people in general feel that there is no value to early detection. There is still a belief that colon surgery will result in a permanent colostomy. Silman and Mitchell (1984) reported that a major barrier to compliance was the nature of the test itself.

Although Simon's review of uncontrolled screening trials showed a range of compliance from 15-98% with most falling in the 50-70% range, he also noted that those programs having high compliance were usually dealing with highly motivated and/or selected groups of subjects. Three studies which carefully documented participant compliance all showed poor results ranging from 22-30% (Simon, 1985).

Macrae et al (1984) found that compliance/acceptance rates were highest in self-selected populations participating in prevention oriented health clinics (80-90%); the next highest in persons approached by their general practitioner (33-45%) and the lowest in persons approached by mail, non-medical volunteers or in groups (5-33%).

Elwood, et al (1978) assessed five different educational approaches to screening for colorectal cancer ranging from impersonal mailings to individual home visits and found an overall compliance of only 15%. Hatfield, (1984) in assessing the effect of colon cancer screening in a large multidisciplinary group practice found the highest level of acceptance if patients were contacted prior to their appointments.

Simon's review of several studies found that the elderly are less compliant with blood stool screening programs than middle aged subjects.

" This is a major weakness of the whole screening concept in that the risk of bowel cancer, the likelihood of a positive test and the predictive

value of positive results all progressively rise
with age, but those individuals most likely to be
helped by screening are paradoxically least
likely to cooperate" (Simon, 1985, p. 830).

Few studies have specifically addressed factors that
affect the use of early detection procedures and programs
in the elderly. Warnecke, et al (1983) stresses the need
for continuity of care and education in the role of early
detection in the elderly and an understanding of the
sociodemographic, behavioral and structural models as
they affect health care patterns in this population.

Health Belief Model indices have resulted in varying
responses when looking at factors affecting compilers and
noncompilers in health screening prorams (Macrae, etal
1984 and Halper, etal 1980). Overall, patient perception
related to symptoms, diseases, body sites and treatment
regimens affect compliance (Halper et al 1980). Macrae
found that the Health Belief Model accounted for 12% of
the variance in screening behavior and that perceived
barriers to taking the test and perceived susceptibility
to bowel cancers were significant.

Another important issue in compliance is the failure of
persons with a positive blood stool result to undergo
workup. Our study found 11% of persons with positive
screens refusing to undergo further workup even after
multiple attempts to encourage them to do so. Other
studies have found as many as 36% of patients with
positive screens lost to follow-up (Simon 1985).

The lack of protocol guidelines, for physicians to
follow, in working up the patients with positive screens
allowed us the opportunity to assess how physicians view
this test and how they evaluate their patients with
occult fecal blood. In 18 cases evaluation was limited
to a repeat blood stool test and only 15 patients
received colonoscopies as part of their workup. This
demonstrates that physician practices in working up
hemocult positive patients varies widely and strategies
to improve public screening programs need to be directed
at physicians as well as the public.

Although the overall results from most screening
programs have been discouraging, successful screening

programs can be achieved with extensive preparation and aggressive public education programs. This requires programs which promote a high level of awareness among both physicians and the public and consequently requires extensive resources, especially manpower, and time to achieve.

COST ANALYSIS

In the absence of convincing demonstration of the efficacy of early detection programs to reduce mortality from colorectal cancer, it is important to assess the costs and benefits of such programs as closely as possible. On first analysis, occult blood screening seems cheap but when one exams the direct and indirect and hidden costs, the few published references to cost appear surprisingly low (Simon 1985).

A great proportion of expense is incurred in the workup and evaluation of false positive results. Using the data from most screening programs, and ours in particular, if 2-6% of screening subjects are hemocult positive, but only 5-10% of these (4% in our study) have cancer, then approximately 2-5% (4% in our study) of all screened subjects will undergo needless followup including expensive tests. (Simon, 1985).

A cost analysis of our two screening programs combined showed direct expenses to run as high as $16,765 (estimates). These direct expenses included the costs of the hemocult kits (provided by the American Cancer Society), fees for follow-up examinations for all positive screened subjects and physician fees.

Indirect expenses are those expenses involved in establishing and running a program. In our program, which relied extensively on volunteer staff, other resource personnel, ie., lab technicians and clerical support, were necessary to support the program. Other indirect expenses included promotion and publicity charges as well as printing and postage fees. The two programs combined had an estimated indirect cost of $26,110. These costs do not factor in administrative time in setting up and overseeing the program.

Hidden costs are not readily apparent and include such elements as patient time and inconvenience, time lost from work, transportation expenses, etc., the emotional costs of undergoing complex procedures, the physical risks from such procedures, a false sense of security in screened negative patients, and the inefficient use of medical resources for the evaluation of false positive results (Simon, 1985). The hidden costs of conducting our program were not estimated.

Cost per participant screened in our study averaged $9.12. Detection of four cancers in the screened population of 4,700 participants cost approximately $43,000 or $10,718 per cancer detected.

TABLE 6. Cost of Colorectal Screening Process *

Direct Expenses	$16,765.00
Indirect Expenses	$26,110.00
Total Expenses	$42,875.00
Number of Cancers Detected	4
Cost per Cancer detected	$10,718.00
Number of participants screened	4,700
Cost per Participant Screened	$ 9.12

* Estimated

This is significantly higher than the $2500 per cancer detected (excluding physician fees) quoted in the other studies (Simon 1985) and suggest that more studies need to look at costs involved in putting on such screening programs.

CONCLUSIONS

Despite emotional arguments in favor of screening for colorectal cancer, little objective evidence is available regarding efficacy. Even simple screening strategies, e.g. stool occult blood testing, are complex and much more costly than generally appreciated.

In this study, 4 malignancies were detected in 92 patients with positive stool occult blood tests. However, thorough evaluation (colonoscopy) was done in only 15 patients and detected 2 cancers. A third and fourth cancer were found at sigmoidoscopy. The 75 other patients may remain at risk. Follow up of this group is planned. The true number of cancers capable of being detected and the cost per case for this method remains unknown.

As stated above, the introduction of a screening program into a community can produce major educational benefits. The intent and purpose of the ACS Colorectal Health Check Program and of this screening in particular was to increase public awareness of colorectal cancer. Attention to risk factors, life style and diet, early detection, warning signs, and treatment options were introduced through this program. Aggressive public education programs do appear to have a more lasting impact on compliance and participation in such programs.

Acknowledgement and thanks to Dia Furber, ART, CTR for the data collection in this project   and to Dr. Herbert Baum for his assistance with the statistical analysis.

REFERENCES

American Cancer Society, Inc (1986). Cancer Facts and Figures, New York.

American Cancer Society, Inc.(1983) Cancer of the Colon and Rectum: Summary of a Public Attitude Survey. CA-A Cancer Journal for Clinicians Vol. 33 No. 6:359-365.

Berwick D M (1985) Screening in Health Fairs: A Critical Review of Benefits, Risks and Costs. JAMA Vol. 254 No.11: 1492-1498.

Dent Owen(1980). Introduction: Physician Awareness of Concepts in Colorectal Cancer. In Winawer S, Schottenfeld D, Sherlock P, (eds): "Colorectal Cancer: Prevention, Epidemiology, and Screening" New York: Raven Press, pp 243-244.

Eddy DM (1981). The Economics of Cancer Prevention and Detection: Getting More for Less.   Cancer 47:1200-1209.

Elwood TW, Erickson PH, Lieberman S (1978). Comparative Educational Approaches to Screening for Colorectal Cancer. AJPH Vol. 68 No. 2: 135-138.

Halper MS, Winawer S, Brody RS, Andrews M, Roth D, a n d
    Burton G (1980). Issues of Patient Compliance. In
    Winawer S, Schottenfeld D, Sherlock P (eds):"Colorectal
    Cancer: Prevention, Epidemiology, and Screening" New
    York: Raven Press, pp 299-310.
Hatfield AK, Bozinovich MA, Steiner JA, Alster JM, Imrey
    PB (1984). Colon Cancer Screening in a Large,
    Multispecialty Group Practice. In "Advances in Cancer
    Control: Epidemiology and Research" New York 156: 283-
Hoffman W (1984). How Worthwhile is Screening for Occult
    Blood? Diagnostic Medicine. May:35-40.
Lefall LD Jr.(1980). Introduction: Factors Influencing
    Patients' Attitudes Toward Screening for Colorectal
    Cancer. In Winawer S, Schottenfeld D, Sherlock P,
    (eds.):"Colorectal Cancer: Prevention, Epidemiology,
and Screening" New York: Raven Press, pp 245-247.
Macrae FA, et al (1984). Preventive Medicine 13: 115-126.
Messner RL, Gardner SS, Webb DD (1986). Early Detection:
    The Priority in Colorectal Cancer. Cancer Nursing 9
    (1): 8-14.
Schottenfeld D, Winawer SJ, (1982). Large Intestine.
    In Schottenfled D, Fraumen J Jr,(eds.):"Cancer
    Epidemiology and Prevention" Philadelphia: WB Saunders
    pp 703-727.
Sherlock P, and Winawer SJ (1977). The Role of Early
    Diagnosis in Controlling Large Bowel Cancer. An
    Overview. Cancer 40: 2609-2615.
Sherlock P,and Winawer SJ (1984) Colorectal Cancer.
    Professional Education, ACS, Inc.
Silman A, Mitchell P (1984). Attitudes of Non-
    Participants in an Occupational Based Programme of
    Screening for Colorectal Cancer. Community Medicine 6:
    8-11.
Simon JB (1985). Occult Blood Screening for Colorectal
    Carcinoma: A Critical Review. Gastroenterology 88:
    820-37.
Warnecke RB, Havelick PL, Manfredi C (1983). Awareness
    and Use of Screening by Older-Aged Persons. In Yancik
    R, et al (eds)." Aging: Perspectives on Prevention and
    Treatment of Cancer in the Elderly" New York: Raven
    Press Vol 24:275-288.
Winawer SJ (1983). Detection and Diagnosis of Colorectal
    Cancer. Cancer 51:2519-2524.
Winawer SJ (1985). Screening for Colorectal Cancer: The
    Issues. Gastroenterology 85:820-37.
Winawer SJ, et al (1980). Progress Report on
    Controlled Trial of Fecal Occult Blood Testing for the
    Detection of Colorectal Neoplasia. Cancer 45:2959-
    2964.

Winawer SJ, Fleisher M, Baldwin M, Sherlock P (1982). Current Status of Fecal Occult Blood Testing in Screening for Colorectal Cancer. CA-A Cancer Journal for Clinicians. Vol. 32 No 2: 100-111.

Winchester DP (1980). A Mass Screening Program for Colorectal Cancer Using Chemical Testing for Occult Blood in the Stool. Cancer 45:2955-2958.

Winchester DP, Sylvester J, Maher ML (1983). Risks and Benefits of Mass Screening for Colorectal Neoplasia with the Stool Guaiac Test. CA-A Cancer Journal for Clinicians. Vol. 33,No. 6:333-343.

Advances in Cancer Control: The War on Cancer—
15 Years of Progress, pages 67–74
© 1987 Alan R. Liss, Inc.

INNOVATIVE APPROACH TO ALTER FATALISTIC MISCONCEPTIONS IN A HIGH CANCER MORTALITY COMMUNITY*

Stephen W. Workman, M.P.H.
Zili Amsel, Sc.D.
Paul F. Engstrom, M.D.

Fox Chase Cancer Center
Philadelphia, PA 19111

Seven misconceptions about cancer were found to be widely held in a population targetted for a community-wide cancer control program. This paper discusses a strategy designed to refute these misconceptions and to prepare the community for further intervention.

The cancer control program is designed to reduce cancer incidence and mortality in a population identified at higher than expected risk. Its goals are (1) to reduce cancer risks by modifying personal habits, and (2) to promote early treatment by encouraging self-surveillance and screening. The program has five principal components:

(1) A community awareness campaign to educate and inform the public.

(2) A self-administered risk assessment form to be distributed throughout the community.

(3) A screening program designed to familiarize the population with detection procedures and to identify early stage illness.

(4) Health education programs to be presented in group settings.

(5) Individual health counseling.

* Supported by NCI-PHS grant #CA34856.

DESCRIPTION OF THE SETTING

The intervention area consists of five adjacent neighborhoods located in a heavily industrialized residential community. According to 1980 census data for the area, 99% of the over 100,000 residents are white. The area is considered working class, and has a median household income of $13,000. Residents of the area are not highly educated; the proportion of high school graduates over the age of 25 is 37.3%, which is significantly below local and national averages. The proportion of college graduates residing in the target area is 3%, also below regional and U.S. averages. (US Bureau of Census, 1980)

The vast majority of local residents have roots in the neighborhood that go back several generations. They are described as tightly knit, maintaining a skeptical view of educational and scientific programs. They are said to be suspicious of the bureaucratic and technical appearance of health-related services. (Childers and Post, 1976) This attitude would appear to be reflected in low rates of response to a baseline survey conducted in anticipation of this study, and to a self-administered risk assessment form which was distributed earlier in the project.

The population has been identified as having a higher than expected risk for cancer mortality. (Dayal et al, 1984) A series of newspaper articles on this topic, published in 1981, helped to increase the community's awareness of the problem. Although it is widely presumed that local industries are responsible for the cancer rate, the Dayal study suggests that personal lifestyle considerations, especially tobacco use, play a decisive role in local cancer incidence. (Dayal, 1984)

IDENTIFICATION OF THE PROBLEM

A health survey questionnaire was undertaken to assess the community's knowledge, practices, and experiences in regard to cancer and heart disease. The questionnaire showed the community to be more aware of cancer than other surveyed populations, yet found respondents largely pessimistic about its ability to be prevented, detected, or treated effectively. (Amsel, et. al., 1984)

A series of focus group interviews was conducted to examine in greater depth the community's attitudes and beliefs about cancer. These interviews proved useful in identifying several misconceptions about cancer, which appear to be widely held by residents of the intervention community:

MISCONCEPTIONS

(1) "There is nothing one can do to prevent cancer"

(2) "There is cancer hidden in everybody; it is a matter of time until it becomes activated"

(3) "Cancer is triggered by a bruise or blow to the body"

(4) "Cancer is inherited"

(5) "Surgery spreads cancer"

(6) "The treatment for cancer is worse than the disease itself"

(7) "Cancer is a death sentence"

The widespread acceptance of these misconceptions within the community is thought to contribute to skepticism about cancer prevention and the value of cancer treatment. This, in turn, would inhibit the adoption of preventive behavior and delay the seeking of treatment.

METHOD

To prepare the community for intervention programs designed to foster the prevention and early detection of cancer, a strategy was developed to refute the seven misconceptions. Specifically, this strategy seeks to replace the misconceptions with accurate information about cancer etiology and treatment, to encourage completion of pre-test and post-test forms, and to motivate the population to participate in additional programs sponsored by the project. Initially, the strategy is directed to women between the ages of 25 and 45 living in the target area. A "Family Centered Communication Model" has been developed to illustrate a

method for establishing contact within the population [FIGURE
I]. In this very traditional community, women are
particularly influential in providing for the health of their
families, overseeing care of their husbands and children, and
often of their parents.

FAMILY CENTERED COMMUNICATIONS MODEL

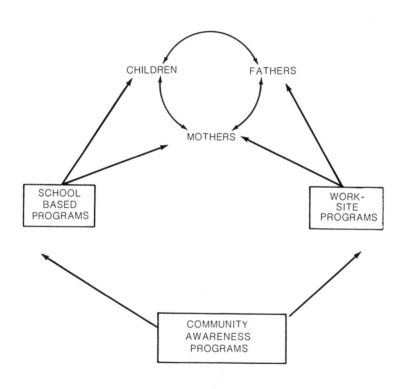

FIGURE I

This strategy is built around two principal components:
a slide/tape program to be presented to parents attending
parent-teacher association meetings, and a classroom program
in which children are given assignments to complete with
their parents. The slide/tape program addresses the parents

directly. The classroom program is designed to reinforce the information provided by the slide/tape program.

This slide/tape program for adults is the centerpiece of the strategy. It is designed to entertain as well as to inform, and it incorporates a pre-test of the audience within its format. Entitled "Beat the Odds," this program takes the form of a television quiz show in which the audience is asked to participate. The first part of the program consists of a series of questions in which participants are asked to agree or disagree with specific statements about the etiology and treatment of cancer. These questions help to prompt audience interest in learning answers to the questions asked, and constitute a pre-test of knowledge and attitudes about cancer. Also included are questions to collect demographic information and to help identify respondents. In the second part of the audio-visual program a physician discusses several facts about cancer, identifying and refuting the misconceptions.

In the classroom intervention program, information about cancer is presented to children in kindergarten through eighth grade. The information presented addresses the misconceptions in a way that the children can understand. The children are encouraged to discuss the presentation at home and are given a handout about cancer "facts and fancies", addressing the misconceptions, which they are asked to take to their parents.

RESEARCH DESIGN

A research design was developed to evaluate both the "Beat the Odds" slide/tape program and the effectiveness of the classroom intervention as a reinforcement tool. Three geographic sub-areas within the target community were selected for the evaluation. These are comparable in terms of numbers of residents, population characteristics, and numbers of schools. Each area contains two parochial schools and one public school.

One of these (area "A") acts as a control area. Its three schools receive neither the "Beat the Odds" slide/tape program nor the classroom intervention. Another classroom program, focusing on the issue of cigarette smoking, is substituted. Following this classroom program, a survey is sent to the parents and collected by the teachers. This

survey constitutes a pre-test of the control area. No
program is offered in place of the adult program in this
control area. Post-test data are gathered six months after
the classroom program is conducted.

The three schools in Area "B" do receive the "Beat the
Odds" program for adults at meetings of their parent-teacher
associations. However, the classroom program is the same one
about cigarette smoking that is offered to children in the
control area. As in the control area, survey forms are sent
to the parents through the schools to provide pre-test
measurements. The pre-test incorporated into the "Beat the
Odds" program is also considered. Once again, post-test
information is gathered six months after conducting the
classroom program.

Area "C" is the only one to receive both components of
the intervention. Parents receive the slide/tape program,
and children receive the intervention classroom program
designed to reinforce it. Pre-test data are collected before
the classroom intervention and at the time of the adult
intervention. Post-test data are gathered six months later.

Thus, data are collected at three points in time for
mothers of children in the intervention areas and at two
points for mothers of children in the control area. In all
three areas the classroom programs serve as mechanisms for
collection of pre-test data. Teachers are asked to encourage
the return of survey forms as a way of attaining a response
rate of at least 75%. Mothers who have more than one child
in school will be asked to return each survey; however only
one survey per household is considered when analyzing pre-
test results. Post-test data are to be gathered in similar
fashion.

RESULTS

To date, the classroom control program has been
presented to children in five schools. A total of 1599
children were given survey forms which were used to pre-test
parents. There were 1168 surveys returned, yielding a return
rate of 73%.

The classroom intervention program has been presented in
two schools with a total population of 857 students. The
surveys in these schools were given to students in advance of

the program; of these, 411 forms were returned, for a response rate of 48%. This rate of response is lower than that of the classroom control program. This may reflect the fact that students were asked to return the forms before they were familiar with the project and before support from the teachers had been elicited. It should be noted that this lower rate of response is still higher than the rates of response to earlier activities associated with the project. The staff is presently considering ways in which personal contact with the teachers may be made before the pre-test forms are sent to the parents in order to improve this response.

"Beat the Odds", the intervention program for adults, has met all objectives for which data are available. To date, it has been presented to parent-teacher association meetings in two schools. A total of 109 adults have attended these programs and fully 100% of parents in attendance returned completed pre-test forms. This is remarkably higher than the response to other surveys conducted in the area and suggests that rates of participation may indeed be increased when a pre-test is incorporated into the format of a program. Evaluations of the program, which were completed by 87% of participants, have described the presentations as entertaining as well as informative. The slide/tape program has also been helpful in drawing forth questions from the audience.

Four presentations of "Beat the Odds" remain to be conducted for completion of the research design. In addition, six month follow-up data, measuring the effects of the program in regard to misconceptions are to be collected through the schools. It is anticipated that these measurements will show the same success as the preliminary results.

REFERENCES

Amsel Z et al, (1986). Heightened awareness among residents of an area experiencing high cancer mortality. Unpublished manuscript, Fox Chase Cancer Center.
Childers T, Post J (1976). The blue collar adult's information needs, seeking behavior and use: Final report. Unpublished manuscript, Drexel University School of Library Science.
Dayal H et al, (1984). Ecologic correlates of cancer

mortality patterns in an industrialized urban population. JNCI 73(3):565-574.

United States Department of Census, Census of Population and Housing, 1980- Summary Tape File 3C.

Advances in Cancer Control: The War on Cancer—
15 Years of Progress, pages 75–92
© 1987 Alan R. Liss, Inc.

WORKER PERCEPTIONS AND ACTIONS TOWARD CANCER
CONTROL IN THE WORKPLACE: AN ANALYSIS OF
BASELINE DATA

Anna P. Schenck, Arnold D. Kaluzny,
Godfrey M. Hochbaum, Rosalind P.
Thomas, Y.Y. Lee, and Thomas C.
Ricketts
Lineberger Cancer Research Center,
University of North Carolina, Chapel
Hill, NC 27514

Louis S. Beliczky, Michael J. Krueger,
and Leslie A. Clegg
Dept. of Industrial Hygiene, United
Rubber Workers International Union,
Akron, OH 44308

BACKGROUND

While the exact number of occupational
cancers as been frequently debated over the last
10 years, it is generally agreed that
approximately 20,000 deaths each year are due to
occupational cancers (Office of Technology
Assessment, 1985). The risks associated with
occupational cancer are not spread evenly across
all work sites or even across all workers within
the same industry. For example, workers in the
rubber industry have been found to have higher
rates of cancers of the lung, colon, blood and
stomach than the general population (Monson and
Nakano, 1976; McMichael, et al., 1976). Looking
specifically at rubber workers, those in certain
work areas such as workers who are exposed to
solvents, are at even greater risk than workers
in other areas. The National Cancer Institute
(NCI) has long been interested in programs which
attempt to reduce the risks of occupational
cancers, most of which are seen as preventable.

Since 1978, NCI has given the Occupational Safety and Health Administration (OSHA) a total of $14 million to add cancer prevention information to the worker training and education activities implemented through OSHA's New Directions programs. In 1983, five unions which had been participating in the New Directions program were awarded NCI grants to evaluate the cancer prevention components of their educational programs. The Industrial Hygiene Department within the International United Rubber, Cork, Linoleum and Plastic Workers of America (hereafter referred to as the URW) was one of the five unions selected for the three year evaluation grant.

The URW decided to name their project LIFE, which stands for "Labor and Industry Focus on Education". To avoid any negative associations with the word "Cancer", the URW decided to focus Project LIFE on the preventive actions workers could take and not solely on the potential disease outcome of cancer. Additionally, since many of the preventive actions of interest, such as use of personal protective equipment, serve to prevent many diseases and injuries other than cancer, the URW Project LIFE was frequently referred to as a health and safety effort, with two general areas of interest: the work place, or health protection component; and the lifestyle, or health promotion component. The preventive actions covered under the health protection component which are of interest to this presentation include: workers' knowledge of the health effects of the chemicals used on their jobs; their use of personal protective equipment; their adherence to recommended personal hygiene practices; and, knowledge and understanding of engineering controls to reduce work place exposures.

The project had three main objectives:

1. To develop, organize and implement model cancer control programs in participating project plants;

2. To evaluate the effectiveness of the programs through the use of a quasi-experimental design; and,
3. To determine the aspects of the industrial organizational environment that affect the implementation and efficacy of the cancer control programs.

METHODOLOGY

Population

The URW has over 400 local unions, with a total membership exceeding 130,000 people. For this study, 24 local unions, representing about 24,000 workers were targeted for study. The selection was designed to include those unions which had been most active in their worker education and training programs and had at least one paid health and safety worker. The 24 unions represent five major rubber corporations and are located across the United States. Two of the smaller local unions are located in the same town and represent the same company. For purposes of this project, they were combined and treated as a single location, leaving 23 project locations.

Project Design

The URW, working with researchers from the University of North Carolina, proposed to evaluate their ongoing cancer prevention programs by introducing an innovative cancer program in some of the locations and comparing the new program to their existing programs. This design required the use of a comparison group. To achieve comparable groups, the following steps, illustrated in Figure 1, were taken.

First, the 23 locations were stratified by company. Then, the plants within each company were paired according to the size of the work force. Ten matched pairs of plants were obtained in this manner. One plant from each pair was randomly assigned to the intervention group, the other plant was designated the comparison group. Of the remaining 3 locations, 2 were assigned to the intervention group. The other was randomly allocated to the intervention group.

FIGURE 1. Project LIFE Design

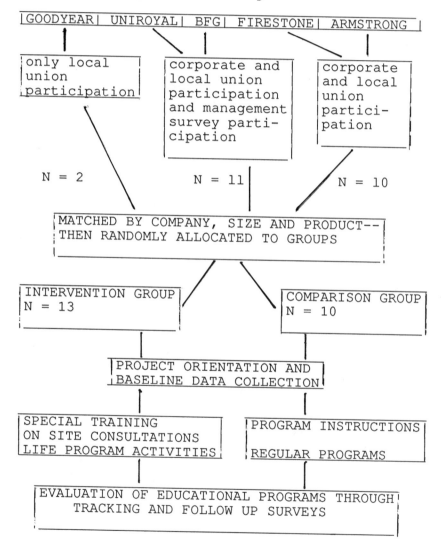

The major evaluation strategy consisted of a self administered questionnaire, implemented at two points in time, before and after the intervention. The intervention phase consisted of training, consultation and program assistance provided to the program implementors.

Sample

Lists of current employees were obtained for each participating location. Based on a need to detect a 15% change, sample size was calculated and randomly selected separately for each location. In September of 1983, 4,689 surveys were mailed to URW workers. Due to the wishes of the local unions that workers' anonymity be protected, no markings were made on the surveys to enable us to track individuals. This fact meant that all promotional materials, by design, had to be generic and not targeted at specific groups who had received the survey. Additionally, follow-up letters had to be sent to all workers in the sample, regardless of whether of not they had completed and returned the survey. Given these constraints, an overall return rate of 35% was achieved, with 1650 completed wage surveys returned. Individual response rates for each location ranged from 18 percent to 50 percent.

TABLE 1. Sample Demographics

Characteristics	Percent
SEX--Male	92%
RACE--White	92%
MARRIED & LIVING WITH SPOUSE	86%
AGE--Under 30	9%
30 -- 34	14%
35 -- 39	17%
40 -- 44	17%
45 -- 49	13%
50 -- 54	14%
55 -- 59	11%
60 and over	5%
YEARS OF SERVICE--0 -- 4	5%
5 -- 9	12%
10 -- 14	20%
15 -- 19	27%
20 -- 24	15%
25 or more	20%
INCOME LEVEL--Under $20,000	10%
$20,000 -- $29,000	61%
$30,000 -- $39,000	26%
$40,000 or more	3%
EDUCATION LEVEL--Less than high school	12%
High school graduation	43%
Post high school educ.	44%

N = 1650

The demographics of the respondents are
presented in Table 1. As can be seen, the study
group is predominantly male (92%), white (92%)
and married (86%). The average respondent is in
the 40-44 age bracket. Eighty-three percent
(83%) have 10 or more years of service with their
companies. The average income level is between
$20-$29,000. As a group, they are better

educated than the general population, with only 12% lacking a high school diploma.

Data Collection Instrument

The baseline survey was a 22 page questionnaire consisting of 145 questions. All surveys were mailed to workers' homes and accompanied by a letter of support from the International Union President. The variables of interest to this session are: workers' knowledge of potential health risks of the chemicals and materials used in their jobs, their use of protective equipment, their use of personal hygiene facilities and their knowledge of the location and operation of engineering controls in their work areas. Additional measures not discussed here include health promotion outcomes such as smoking cessation, exercise, nutrition awareness and stress reduction.

BASELINE DATA

Knowledge of Health Effects of Chemicals

OSHA regulates 1300 known hazardous chemicals in the work place. There are over 10,000 chemicals used in the rubber industry and estimates about the number of chemicals which are suspected or known health threats vary widely. To assess rubber workers' knowledge of the potentially hazardous nature of the substances with which they work, respondents were asked whether or not they worked with chemicals which they thought might pose a threat to their health. This question was intended simply as a screening question, to allow those whose jobs did not involve chemicals to skip the more specific questions. However, 22% of the respondents indicated that they were not sure whether the chemicals they used on their jobs posed a threat to their health. As a follow up question, respondents were also asked: "How informed do you think you are about the health effects of the chemicals and materials you work with?" The response options were: very informed, moderately informed, somewhat informed and not at all informed. Only 6% of the respondents indicated they were very informed. Overall, the results indicate that 24% of the respondents felt very informed or moderately informed. Both of these figures exclude the 22% who were instructed to skip the question because they were not sure about the health effects of their work chemicals. Furthermore, the proportion of workers who report they are well informed varies by company.

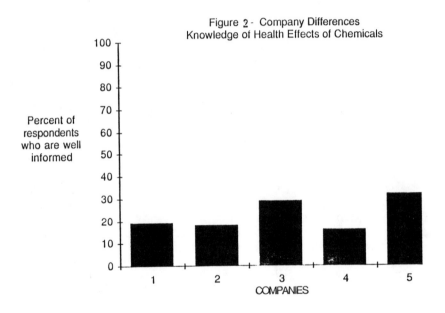

Figure 2 - Company Differences
Knowledge of Health Effects of Chemicals

Percent of respondents who are well informed

COMPANIES

Chi-square = 23.849

d.f. = 4

Overall n = 966

As can be seen in Figure 2, the company percentages of respondents indicating they felt well informed varied from a high of 32% to a low of 16% (chi-square = 23.849,p=0.0001).

Knowledge of Location and Operation of Engineering Controls

There are three basic types of engineering controls which are use to reduce rubber workers exposure to potentially harmful substances: enclosed systems for storage and transfer of chemicals; local exhaust ventilation and the use of bagged materials. Again, as a screening question, we asked respondents whether any of the above types of controls were used in their work areas. Ten percent indicated they were not sure if any such controls were used in their work areas. Respondents who answered that controls were used in their work areas were asked how informed they thought they were about the location and operation these engineering controls. Again, the response options were: very, moderately, somewhat or not at all informed. The overall percentage of respondents who indicated they were very or moderately informed was 47%. However, the overall score masks important company differences. As shown in Figure 3, company responses ranged from 59% to 37% (chi-square = 20.047, p=0.0005).

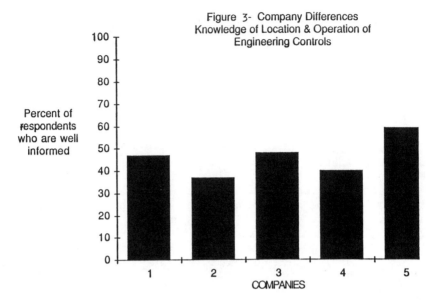

Figure 3- Company Differences Knowledge of Location & Operation of Engineering Controls

Chi-square = 20.047

d.f. = 4

Overall n = 964

While the percentages of respondents who reported they were well informed about engineering controls were much higher than those for chemical awareness, these results must be looked at in light of the large number of respondents (1/3) who indicated that such a question was not applicable their work areas. Thus, while workers may be better informed about engineering controls *when they exist*, a large proportion of the work force believe they have no such controls.

Use of Separate Lockers for Work and Home Clothes

Standard accepted personal hygiene practices for rubber workers include the use of separate lockers for work and street clothes, so that dusts and potentially harmful materials are not carried into workers' homes. Overall, 84% of the respondents indicated they always or usually use the lockers as recommended. However, as with many other protective procedures, responses to this question varied between companies. As shown in Figure 4, the percentage of respondents who complied with the locker recommendation ranged from 94% to 79% (chi-square = 43.763, p = 0.0001).

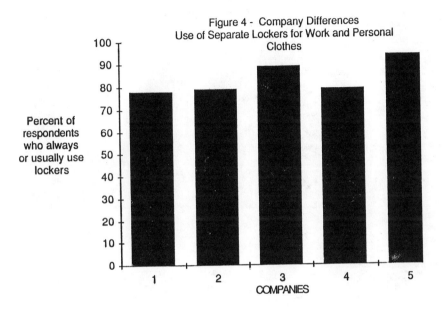

Figure 4 - Company Differences
Use of Separate Lockers for Work and Personal Clothes

Chi-square = 43.763

   d.f. = 4

Overall n = 1485

Use of Showers

Another recommended personal hygiene practice for rubber workers is to shower after work before going home; again, to avoid inadvertently transferring the work chemicals into the home environment. Overall, 57% of the respondents who have work showers available indicated they always or usually use them as recommended. As shown in Figure 5, company responses varied, ranging from 67% to 28% (chi=square = 95.591, p=0.0001).

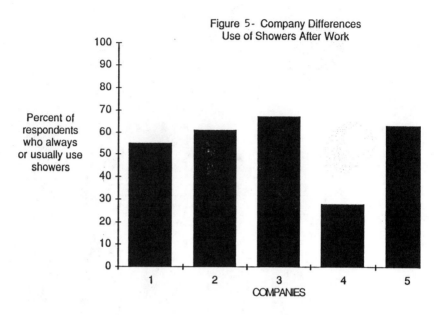

Figure 5- Company Differences
Use of Showers After Work

Chi-square = 95.591

d.f. = 4

Overall n = 1466

Eating or Drinking in the Work Areas

Accepted work practices in the rubber industry call for workers to refrain from eating or drinking while in the work areas, to avoid the possibility of having chemicals and particles from the rubber processes settle on their food. When asked how frequently they ate or drank in their work areas, less than half (48%) of the respondents indicated they rarely ate or drank in their work areas. As can be seen in Figure 6, looking at the responses by company reveals a range from 59% to 33% (chi-square = 55.516, p = 0.0001).

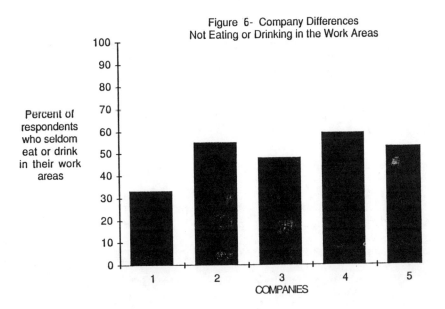

Figure 6- Company Differences
Not Eating or Drinking in the Work Areas

Chi-square = 55.516

d.f. = 4

Overall n = 1580

Perceived Effectiveness at Protecting the Health of Workers

Certainly no one group of people alone can solve the health and safety issues facing industrial workers. It will take many groups, including workers, their unions and management joined in cooperative efforts to deal with the health and safety challenge. How effective the responsible groups are perceived to be will be very important in their ability to work cooperatively. When asked to rate the effectiveness of several groups at protecting workers from occupational health problems, the following results were observed:

TABLE 2. Overall Effectiveness Ratings of
Responsible Groups

Groups	% Rating High Effectiveness*
1. Health & safety committees	42%
2. International union officials and dept. of industrial hygiene	35%
3. Co-workers	34%
4. Local plant management	25%
5. Company headquarters	18%

*Includes those who rated the groups as quite or very effective.

N = 1549

As can be seen in Table 2, the health and safety committees were the group most frequently considered "quite" or "very" effective, followed by the International union industrial hygiene officials and co-workers. Surprisingly, the two groups who might be expected to have the greatest policy impact on the protection of workers' health and safety, the local plant management and the company headquarters, were viewed by the workers as the least effective. While these data cannot attest to the actual effectiveness of management and company headquarters, the low perceived effectiveness is likely to hamper any efforts on their part to implement actions or programs which improve work related safety and health.

TABLE 3. Mean Effectiveness Ratings of
Responsible Groups by Company

Groups

Company	H&S Comm	Int'l Union	Co-Workers	Local Mgmt	Co. HQ
1	3.45	3.32	3.14	3.03	2.78
3	3.38	3.21	3.05	2.91	2.66
5	3.31	3.01	3.12	2.89	2.57
2	3.05	2.97	2.92	2.42	2.28
4	2.99	2.85	2.90	2.68	2.57

Overall N = 1549

When the mean effectiveness ratings for each
group are compared across companies, two
interesting observations emerge which can be seen
in Table 3. First, the pattern seen earlier,
with the health and safety committees receiving
the highest ratings and company headquarters
receiving the lowest, is consistent across all 5
companies. Secondly, although the pattern across
groups is consistent, three of the companies have
means which are significantly higher than the
other two companies. Using one way ANOVA and
Scheffe's multiple comparison test, companies 2
and 4 were always shown to have significantly
lower effectiveness ratings than companies 1, 3,
and 5.

CONCLUSIONS

As demonstrated by the data presented here,
there are a number of cancer control practices in
the rubber industry that could be more adequately
implemented. First, and most basic, is the need
to improve workers' knowledge concerning the
chemicals and materials with which they work. In

1980, the Department of Health and Human Services (DHHS) issued the following objective:

By 1990, at least 25% of workers should be able, *prior to employment*, to state the nature of their occupational health and safety risks and their potential consequences...(US Dept. Health and Human Services, 1980).

Despite this objective, as seen in these data, workers, the majority of whom have been employed an average of 10 years, are unable to state the nature of their occupational health risks. Without understanding of the nature of the health risks involved in their work, it will be difficult to make many of the other needed changes to improve workers' safety and health. The OSHA Federal Hazardous Substances Communication Standard recently implemented requires employers to provide workers with training on the chemicals used in their work areas. This standard should help increase the level of awareness among workers.

However, increased awareness by itself is not likely to lead to adoption of many of the recommended protective actions. Many barriers exist making it difficult for workers to consistently adhere to recommended practices. Reasons for the low compliance with recommended behaviors are varied but can be illustrated by the following comments typically heard at the local plants:

"To use the showers often means a wait in a line at the end of a long shift", or, "the showers are not in good working order";

"To eat only in the enclosed break areas often means using half of the break walking to and from the area";

"To use protective equipment makes it difficult to do a job and still make production demands, and the equipment is often uncomfortable or unavailable."

In addition to the barriers just listed, the challenge of cancer control in the work place is further complicated by the differing nature of the processes, management styles, work regulations and engineering controls between companies.

One message from these data is clear--there is much to be done in the work place to reduce cancer risks. It is evident that existing programs have not eliminated the problem and that new strategies tailored to the specific work conditions are needed.

Project LIFE is currently testing several new cancer control strategies. In addition to the data presented here, information about why workers did not adhere to recommended practices and their beliefs about the effectiveness of such practices were collected. Plant specific information was discussed with local program contacts, who were provided training, consultation and program assistance in attempts to implement programs which addressed concerns specific to each location.

Results of the Project LIFE program are not yet known. Preliminary observations indicate that while this approach is working very well in some locations, in others, it was not implemented, despite specific training efforts. Data from this project will help us understand not only which program strategies work best, but under what conditions.

This study was supported by funds made available by the URCLPW of A, AFL-CIO through a grant funded by NCI's Occupational Cancer Branch (1-RO1-CA34912-01).

REFERENCES

McMichael AJ, Spirtas R, Gamble JF and Tousey PM
    (1976). Mortality Among Rubber Workers:
    Relationship to Specific Jobs. Journal of
    Occupational Medicine 18(3):178-185.
Monson R and Nakano K (1976). Mortality Among
    Rubber Workers. American Journal of
    Epidemiology 10:284-295.
Office of Technology Assessment (1985).
    "Preventing Illness and Injury in the
    Work place." Washington, DC.
U.S. Department of Health and Human Services
    Public Health Service (1980). "Promoting
    Health/Preventing Disease: Objectives for
    The Nation." US Government Printing Office,
    Washington, DC.

Advances in Cancer Control: The War on Cancer—
15 Years of Progress, pages 93–100
© 1987 Alan R. Liss, Inc.

WORKSITE SMOKING CESSATION: A TEST OF TWO PROGRAMS

Beti Thompson, Ph.D.[1], Gilbert Omenn, M.D.,
Ph.D.[1,2], Mary Sexton, Ph.D.,M.P.H.[3], Bryce
Breitenstein, M.D.,M.P.H.[4], Nancy Hessol,
M.S.P.H.[4], Susan Curry, Ph.D.[1], Marie Michnich,
Dr.P.H.[2], Arthur Peterson, Ph.D.[1,2].

[1] Fred Hutchinson Cancer Research Center, 1124
Columbia, Seattle, WA 98104. [2] School of Public
Health, University of Washington, Seattle, WA
98195. [3] Department of Epidemiology, University
of Maryland Medical School, Baltimore, MD 21201.
[4] Hanford Environmental Health Foundation,
Richland, WA 99352.

Smoking continues to have significant and detrimental
effects on morbidity and mortality (Loeb, et al, 1984;
Phillips et al, 1985). Despite the overwhelming evidence
of the adverse health effects associated with smoking,
approximately 30% of adults in this country continue to
smoke (Lambert et al, 1982; USDHHS, 1979). When
questioned about their habit, 70% to 90% of smokers say
they would like to stop smoking (USDHHS, 1979).
Furthermore, many smokers believe they need assistance in
achieving cessation (USDHHS, 1981).

Many ways have been developed to assist smokers to
achieve cessation; one of these, which has the potential
of reaching large numbers of smokers, is cessation
programs at the worksite (Institute of Med., 1981;
Stachnik et al, 1983). Worksite intervention is
desirable for a number of reasons: (1) worksites have
available, defined populations; (2) efforts can be
directed toward specific groups; for example, blue collar
workers who are disproportionately represented in the
smoking population, may be specifically targeted through
a worksite intervention; (3) worksite interventions offer
the advantage of convenience for employees, especially

when classes, materials, and/or support groups are available at the worksite and at times around working hours; and finally, (4) the benefits of smoking cessation are experienced by both the employer and employees, providing incentives to implement and participate in worksite programs.

Few studies have attempted smoking cessation intervention at large worksites. Furthermore, there is evidence that smoking cessation intervention at large worksites is different from similar interventions at smaller worksites (Fielding, 1985; USDHHS, 1985). In this study, we collaborated with a large worksite in Southeastern Washington State. The worksite employs approximately 14,000 people among nine different contractors. All contractors endorsed this project. The worksite requires annual medical examinations and keeps records of all employees and smoking data from these records were made available to us. Thus, we could determine smoking prevalence at the worksite and gain additional information on the composition of our population.

Our research objectives at the worksite were two-fold:

1. To determine the relative effectiveness of two state-of-the-art smoking cessation programs within a large worksite setting; and

2. To integrate the most effective program into the ongoing health promotion activities at the worksite.

The two programs used are similar in some respects. They are both multi-component, and focus on skills-training, behavior modification, negative reinforcement, stress management, and weight control.

There are some differences between the programs. The MCP, Multiple Components Program, is a proprietary program which focuses on initial cessation. It requires a relatively short time period. Program participants meet once to prepare for quitting, undergo, during the next week, an intensive quit period for four consecutive days in which they are encouraged to quit abruptly, "cold turkey"; then meet once the following week to reinforce the cessation. The program is didactic, with participants listening to lectures, watching slides, or listening to tapes throughout the program sessions.

The RPP, Relapse Prevention Program, was developed specifically to focus on relapse prevention. It requires a longer time period; participants meet weekly for a period of eight weeks. The emphasis is not on immediate quit; rather, participants are allowed to choose an immediate or a phased quit, which may include a cutting down period. The program is interactive, with participants and facilitators sharing experiences and problems encountered along the way.

The programs were offered in two modalities: a group-help modality in which facilitators met with participants in small group sessions; and a self-quit modality, in which participants received written materials and other aids to assist them in their cessation effort. We gave our control groups a minimal intervention consisting of widely available smoking cessation written materials.

In order to maximize the number of smokers we could assist, we used a company-wide survey to identify smokers and ascertain their interest in quitting. Surveys were mailed to employees at their work addresses and were returned via internal worksite mail. One follow-up was made to non-respondents. Responses were received from 9,461 employees for a total response rate of 71%. Of the respondents, 1,743 were current smokers and 79% of those smokers indicated interest in quitting (see Table 1).

TABLE 1
Respondents to Health Promotion Survey

	N	%	
Respondents	9,461	71	
Never Smoked	4,901	52	(of
Ex-smokers	2,683	28	respondents)
Smokers	1,743	18	
Interested in Quitting	1,369	79	(of smokers)

After a short pilot indicated high post-randomization drop-out due to preference for a specific modality (i.e., group-quit or self-quit), smokers were given the opportunity to select their modality of choice and some options as to class times and locations. The preference survey showed that nearly half of the respondents preferred a self-quit modality (48.4%), with a smaller percentage having no preference, and an even smaller percentage preferring a group-quit modality (see Table 2).

TABLE 2
Preference Survey Results

Preference	N	%
Group Preference	126	14.9
Self Preference	410	48.4
No Preference	226	26.6
Other	86	10.1
Total	848	100

Since evidence suggests that smokers tend to do better in group-quit formats, we assigned all those with no preference to the group-quit modality. Smokers were then sent invitations to participate. These were sent to their work addresses. The invitation included a baseline questionnaire, an informed consent form, and instructions to go to a worksite medical aid station. At the aid stations, medical personnel randomized smokers to MCP, RPP, or control within their modality of choice. Those who preferred or were assigned to group-quit were registered for a class at the aid station; and self-quit participants were given their materials.

This system of registration and information dissemination was very easy to implement. Aid station personnel received a one session training period in which the protocol was discussed and questions answered. Aid station personnel indicated that the process was only minimally disruptive to their daily routine.

Participants will be followed for a full year; as of March, 1986, they have completed their six month follow-up. The results are summarized in Table 3.

TABLE 3
Quit Rates by Program Type

Program	Follow-up One (Initial)	Follow-up Two (3 Months)	Follow-up Three (6 Months)
	Percent Quit		
Group			
MCP	61.0	37.3	39.2
RPP	36.8	29.8	28.1
Control	11.8	11.8	11.8
Self			
MCP	18.4	15.8	19.7
RPP	12.2	12.2	15.8
Control	8.2	11.8	12.9

Within the group-quit modality, the MCP showed very high initial cessation rates (61% of those randomized to that program). This compares with 36.8% for the RPP program and 11.8% for the controls. By the three month follow-up, however, the sustained cessation rates for the MCP group have dropped considerably, down to 37.3%, compared to a smaller drop in RPP to 29.8% and a stable level for the control group. The six month follow-up shows very little change from the three month follow-up.

Within the self-quit modality, the MCP program again shows higher initial quit with a drop-off by the three month follow-up. At six months, all three of the self-quit arms show an increase in cessation. We are continuing analysis of this to determine if these are "new" quitters or relapsers who quit again.

Chi-squared tests of the various comparison groups show that, for all follow-ups within the group-quit modality, either program is better than the minimal program offered to the control group (see Table 4).

TABLE 4

Comparisons of Quit Rates by Programs

Comparison	Follow-up One (Initial)	Follow-up Two (3 Months)	Follow-up Three (6 Months)
	P Value		
Group			
Program vs. Control	<.001	.019	.02
MCP vs. Control	<.001	.009	.01
RPP vs. Control	.005	.11	.10
MCP vs. RPP	.02	.33	.53
Self			
Program vs. Control	.17	.60	.33
MCP vs. Control	.11	.31	.29
RPP vs. Control	.49	.99	.63
MCP vs. RPP	.50	.33	.74

Initially, MCP is better than RPP, but by three months, that difference is no longer significant. By the three month follow-up, the difference between RPP and control is no longer significant. Within the self-help modality, there are no significant differences between programs and control or between programs.

We are continuing our analysis to explore the characteristics associated with quitting. Preliminary results show that smoking history, number of prior quit attempts, age, and gender are associated with successful cessation.

A number of conclusions may be derived from these preliminary results of this study.

1. Special research tactics may be needed at the worksite. We found the employees were reachable, but that it was important to build the intervention around worksite locations, appropriate times, and the wishes of the employees. This required us to modify our design.

2. It is possible to reach large numbers of people. We knew, based on the employee medical records that there were 3,769 smokers at that worksite. The smokers who expressed interest in quitting numbered 1,369. We randomized 402 smokers. This was 29% of those interested, and 10.7% of the smoking population at the worksite.

3. As far as the test of the program is concerned, in group-quit formats MCP works better for initial cessation, but by three months, the differences are no longer significant.

4. In self-quit formats, no significant differences were found between programs.

The question of which program or programs to integrate into the worksite has not yet been resolved. While our follow-up continues, the worksite has elected to use the MCP program in group format for those who want a group-quit. Although no difference is significant past initial cessation, personnel argue that the program is easier to implement (though more costly) and more satisfactory to participants. Our data also suggest that quitting is a process, with the majority of smokers requiring more than one successful quit attempt to achieve a sustained quit. From that perspective, the program which maximizes initial cessation may be most effective in the long run if combined with periodic reinforcement.

Further investigation of variables related to successful cessation, as well as descriptions of those who chose not to participate, those who dropped out of the programs, and reactions to the programs continues and will contribute to the final recommendation as to which program should be integrated into ongoing health promotion activities of the worksite.

References:

Fielding JE (1985). Smoking: health effects and control (part 2). N Engl J Med 313: 555–561.

Institute of Medicine (1981). Evaluating health promotion in the workplace. Washington D.C.: National Academy Press.

Lambert CA, Vetherton DR, Finison LF, (1982). Risk factors and life style: a statewide health interview survey. N Engl J Med 306 (17): 1048–51.

Loeb LA, Ernster VL, Warner KE, Abbots J, Laszlo J.
   (1984) Smoking and lung cancer: An overview. Cancer
   Res 44:5940–5958.
Phillips B, Marshall ME, Brown S, Thompson JS (1985).
   Effect of smoking on human natural killer cell
   activity. Cancer 56:2789–2792.
Stachnik TS, Stoffelmayr B (1983). Worksite smoking
   cessation programs: a potential for national impact.
   Am J Publ Health 73 (12): 1395–1396.
U.S. Dept. Health and Human Services (1979). Healthy
   People: The Surgeon General's Report on Smoking and
   Health. Washington, D.C. U.S. Government Printing
   Office.
U.S. Dept. Health and Human Services (1981). The
   Changing Cigarettes: A Report of the Surgeon General.
   Washington, D.C.: U.S. Government Printing Office.
U.S. Department Health and Human Services (1985). The
   Health Consequences of Smoking: Cancer and Chronic
   Lung Disease in the Workplace: A Report of the Surgeon
   General. Washington, D.C.: U.S. Government Printing
   Office.

Advances in Cancer Control: The War on Cancer—
15 Years of Progress, pages 101–108
© 1987 Alan R. Liss, Inc.

SMOKING POLICY AT THE WORKSITE: EMPLOYEE REACTIONS TO
POLICY CHANGES

Beti Thompson, Ph.D.*, Mary Sexton Ph.D.**, Jan
Sinsheimer, M.S.*

*Fred Hutchinson Cancer Research Center, 1124
Columbia, Seattle, WA 98104. **Department of
Epidemiology, University of Maryland Medical
School, Baltimore, Maryland 21201

Many employers are concerned with the adverse effects
of smoking on both their smoking and non-smoking
employees. In addition to the obvious health costs,
economic costs associated with smoking at the workplace
include higher insurance rates, higher absenteeism rates,
and lower productivity (Kristein, 1983; Bennet et al,
1980). A further concern of employers is litigation by
non-smoking employees who demand the right to work in a
smoke-free environment (Garland et al, 1985). For these
reasons, many employers find it appealing to institute a
company-wide restrictive smoking policy. For some
employers, however, a worksite policy is suspect; fears
that smoking employees may sue the company and
difficulties in implementing and enforcing a policy are
some reasons cited for reluctance to implement
restrictive smoking policies (Weiss, 1984; HRPC, 1985).
Another commonly cited objection is the effect on
employee morale (Bennet et al, 1980; HRPC, 1985).

Few studies have looked specifically at the reactions
of employees to new smoking restrictions at the worksite
(Weiss, 1984). The purpose of this study is to provide
more detailed information concerning employee reaction to
a smoking policy. Specifically, the effect of smoking
status on employee reactions is examined. Other
variables, including education, stress, gender, age,
health practices, and smoking history are also examined
for their relationship to employee reactions. In this
paper, we present preliminary results from this project.

Methods

A high-tech company in the Pacific Northwest
instituted a new company-wide restrictive smoking policy
in June, 1985. The policy restricts smoking to only a
few designated areas in the company cafeterias. The
company collaborated with the researchers to conduct a
company-wide survey of employees at the time the
restrictive smoking policy was implemented. The entire
9,019 employee work force was surveyed with an "Employee
Health Survey" which was developed for the project. The
survey included items on health practices, health
promotion at the worksite, reactions to the new policy,
smoking practices, and sociodemographic items. Surveys
were disseminated to employees via their immediate
supervisors, if appropriate, or internal plant mail. No
follow-up of non-respondents was conducted.

Results

Of the 9,019 employees, 4,955 responded for a 55%
response rate. Characteristics of the respondents are
summarized in Table 1. Only 17.5% of respondents are
smokers; this probably reflects differences in survey
response rates rather than actual smoking prevalence
rates at this worksite.

TABLE 1
Respondents to Health Promotion Survey

Characteristics	N	%
Gender		
Male	2,507	52.2
Female	2,368	47.3
Education		
Less than high school	165	3.3
High school graduate	942	19.0
Some college	2,020	40.8
College graduate	842	17.0
Some graduate work	432	8.7
Graduate degree	520	10.5
Smoking Status		
Never smoked	2,663	53.7
Former smoker	1,193	24.1
Current smoker	865	17.5
Age $\bar{X} = 38.1$		

Reactions to the current smoking policy are summarized in Table 2. The majority of respondents were in favor of the new policy.

TABLE 2
Reactions to Smoking Policy

Reaction	N	%
In favor	3,449	69.6
Don't care	841	17.0
Opposed	485	9.8

Those who opposed the policy were more likely to be smokers (see Figure 1). In addition, former smokers were more likely to be opposed than non-smokers.

FIGURE 1

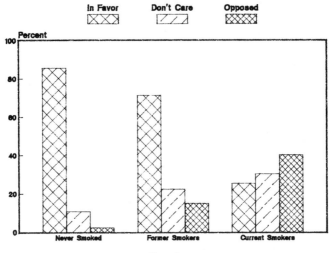

**Reaction to Restrictive Smoking Policy
By Smoking Status**

An examination of characteristics of current smokers by their reactions to the policy (see Figure 2) showed that women, heavier smokers, those who have been smoking for a longer time, those who report fewer health practices, and older respondents were more likely to oppose the policy.

FIGURE 2

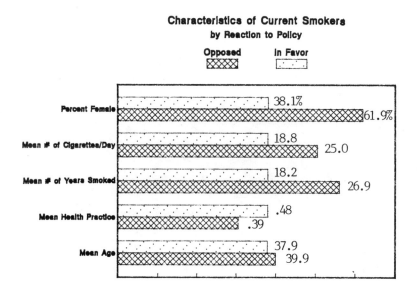

Characteristics of Current Smokers
by Reaction to Policy

Opposed   In Favor

There were differences among "former smokers" in their reaction to the policy (see Figure 3). Length of time smoked and time since quit were associated with negative reactions to the policy.

FIGURE 3

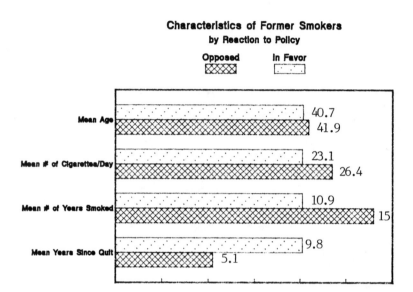

Characteristics of Former Smokers
by Reaction to Policy

A discriminant analysis was conducted to examine the reactions of current smokers to the policy. The results are summarized in Table 3.

TABLE 3

Discriminant Analysis of Current Smokers
and Reactions to Policy

Function: OPREST = PROB + CDAY + WANTQT
          + HEALTH + CONFID + SEX + AGE

Wilks' Lambda = .792
R^2 = .208
Percent correctly classified = 68.7%

Step	Variable Entered	Correlation with Function
1	PROB, probability of quitting	.319
2	CDAY, cigarettes per day	−.497
3	WANTQT, desire to quit	.386
4	HEALTH, health practices	.397
5	CONFID, confidence in quitting	.219
6	SEX, gender	.189
7	AGE, age	−.141

Variables not entered into the analysis include:
education, stress, and total time smoked.

From the discriminant analysis, two additional
characteristics of those smokers most likely to be
opposed to the policy were identified; these include
those who have little desire to quit, and those who have
little perceived probability of quitting.

A discriminant analysis of former smokers and their
reactions did not improve classifications and yielded a
small R^2.

Conclusions

The most significant finding of this study is that, overall, only a small minority of employees is opposed to a restrictive worksite smoking policy. Current smokers are much more likely to object than never-smokers or former smokers. Those smokers most likely to object are female, older smokers who smoke more, have smoked longer, have fewer current health practices, and have less desire to quit. This is congruent with other findings.

Because of the generally favorable attitudes toward a smoking policy, employers, in the interest of reducing health hazards and also for economic reasons, should be encouraged to implement policies which restrict smoking at the workplace.

References:

Bennet D, Levy BS, (1980). Smoking policies and smoking cessation programs of large employers of Massachusetts. Am J Publ Health 70 (6): 629-631.

Garland C, Barett-Connor E, Suarez L, Criqui MH, Wingard DL (1985). Effects of passive smoking on ischemic heart disease mortality of nonsmokers. Am J Epidemiol 121 (5): 645-650.

Human Resources Policy Corporation (1985). Smoking Policies in Large Corporations. Los Angeles: Human Resources Policy Corporation.

Kristein MM (1983). How much can business expect to profit from smoking cessation. Prev Med 12:358-381.

Weis, WL (1984). No smoking. Pers J Sept: 53-58.

Advances in Cancer Control: The War on Cancer—
15 Years of Progress, pages 109–119
© 1987 Alan R. Liss, Inc.

CANCER EDUCATION AND SCREENING IN THE WORKPLACE: THE CORPORATE PERSPECTIVE

L. Zimmerman, M.P.H., G. Jackson, M.D.
J. Hughes, M.D., M. Minkoff
Kelsey-Seybold Foundation's
Cancer Prevention Center
6624 Fannin, Houston, Texas 77030

INTRODUCTION

The Kelsey-Seybold Foundation was established in Houston by physicians and community leaders at the Kelsey-Seybold Clinic in 1956 to provide financial support for specific projects in clinical or basic science medical research and education.

In 1983 the Foundation received two major gifts from supporters, Joe and Jessie Crump and Joseph and Madelyn Vercellino, to form the Cancer Prevention Center.

The Cancer Prevention Center focuses on the early detection and prevention of breast and colon cancers through screening, service to the community, education and cancer research in collaboration with scientists from other teaching institutions in the Texas Medical Center. The goal of the Cancer Prevention Center is to bring the newest methods of early detection to the Houston community, while expanding knowledge about cancer prevention and cure.

Current projects include:

* A comprehensive cancer awareness program for company employees.

* Cancer prevention through patient education and lifestyle alteration.

* Screening examination for cancers where early detection offers the best hope of cure.

In 1984, the Pennzoil Company pledged $350,000.00 over a five-year period to the Kelsey-Seybold Foundation and the University of Texas' M.D. Anderson Hospital for a joint research effort aimed at early detection and prevention of cancer.

As a follow-up to its grant, in 1985 Pennzoil assisted the Cancer Prevention Center in developing a model Cancer Awareness and Screening Program for company employees.

This changed the Cancer Prevention Center and made it unique in that it could offer a complete and thorough program of education, consultation, screening, examination and research for a select corporate population.

The Pennzoil Cancer Awareness Program was designed as a component of the company's wellness program. The purpose of the Cancer Awareness Program is to increase health awareness among employees, and to detect cancer in its early stages when the chances of being cured are high.

To underscore his interest in achieving high participation, in the Cancer Awareness Program, Pennzoil President Dr. Richard J. Howe agreed to have Pennzoil cover the cost for the initial screening and testing for all employees and spouses.

Currently, Pennzoil's program focuses on screening for breast and colorectal cancer; later, it may be expanded to include other types of cancer.

The design of the Cancer Awareness Program was a comprehensive three-part program. Stage one of the program consists of a 30-minute presentation of general information about cancer, its causes, prevention and detection, by doctors from Kelsey-Seybold's Cancer Prevention Center. After the presentation, each employee is asked to fill out a risk assessment form designed by the American Cancer Society. These forms are collected by Cancer Prevention Center staff members who review the forms and notify each employee of the results.

Employees whose scores on the risk assessment indicate that they may be at risk are encouraged to participate in stage two of the program. Participants in stage two are given a more detailed questionnaire which they are asked to complete at home. The questionnaire is then mailed to the Cancer Prevention Center for analysis.

Participation in the program is entirely voluntary and completely confidential. Employees mail their questionnaires directly to the Cancer Prevention Center where they are analyzed by doctors and nurses who respond in writing to the employee's home address. Pennzoil sees only summary data relating to participation, cancer detections, and demographic information.

If the analysis of the detailed questionnaire by the Cancer Prevention Center staff indicates that the employee should undergo further testing or screening, this is reflected in the response to the employee. The employee then decides whether he or she wants to participate in the testing or screening. If he/she elects to do so, the initial consultation with the nurse educator, and a mammogram, hemoccult, or short colonoscopy, is paid for by Pennzoil.

The Cancer Awareness lectures were presented twice weekly by Kelsey-Seybold Foundation Cancer Prevention Center physicians at Pennzoil. Each department at Pennzoil Place was scheduled a date and lecture to attend by the Employee Health Nurses. Posters designed by Pennzoil's Community Relations Department were placed in employee coffee rooms, restrooms, and at elevators on each floor. Make-up lectures were scheduled for employees who could not attend their group's lectures. If an employee missed the appointed lecture, the employee received a memo from the President of Pennzoil Company strongly urging attendance at the next make-up session. Thus, strong support for the program came from the top management and encouraged participation among all levels of employees at Pennzoil.

PENNZOIL DEMOGRAPHICS

Figure 1

PENNZOIL COMPANY

DEMOGRAPHIC DATA

AGE	MALE	FEMALE	TOTAL
40-69	308*	134*	442*
35-49	111	122*	233
20-34	360	471	831
TOTAL	779	727	1506

* Appropriate to include in screening catagory due to age.

July 1985

Approximately 1500 of the 7300 Pennzoil employees are housed at the Pennzoil Place Headquarters in Houston. 51% of these are male; 49% female, ranging in ages from 20 to 69 years of age. 39.5% of the males were age 40 or over, qualifying them for the Cancer Awareness Program screening. Similarly 35.2% of the women were age

35 and older, qualifying them for baseline mammograms and breast exams.

Of the 1506 employees officed at Pennzoil Place, 87.3%, or 1314 individuals participated in the Cancer Awareness Program.

Figure 2

PENNZOIL STATISTICS

TOTAL NUMBER OF EMPLOYEES AT PRESENTATIONS - 1,314

Female = 55%
Male = 45%

Category	Male	Female	Total #
high risk consults needed	236	298	534
mammograms			123
short colono-scopies*			123

*Some women require 2 consults, since they are at high risk for both

All 1314 attended the lectures and filled out the initial American Cancer Society Risk Assessment Form. 534 of these individuals, or 40% were found to be at moderate risk based on age, family history, personal medical history or symptoms.

There were approximately 236 men and 298 women. 123 or 32% of those men and women identified as at risk followed up with flexible fiberoptic colon examinations. Similarly, 49%, or 123, of the women identified as being at risk followed through with breast examinations and/or mammograms. Of the 123 colonoscopies performed, 22 polyps were found, 15 were hyperplastic and seven were adenomatous. Of the mammograms completed, three were found to be suspicious but required no biopsies. Given the compliance and participation rate of employee screening programs noted in the literature, the level of participation for Houston based Pennzoil employees was commendable.

This program that educated 87% of the Houston based employess, boosted company morale, and potentially prevented some cancers, cost Pennzoil approximately, $55,800.00 or $42.46 per participating employee. In employee benefit terms in Houston, this approximates the per person cost of a Christmas Party and company picnic-neither of which have the personal impact of this program.

Thus, Pennzoil is pleased. The cost of the Cancer Awareness Program can, from a corporate perspective, also be analyzed.

It has been stated many times over, that although there is an initial dollar expenditure for the programs, health awareness and health promotion programs save industry large amounts of money in insurance premiums, employee absenteeism, and associated costs. Annually, this can amount to over $10 Billion dollars. (Page and Asire, 1985; Eddy, 1981)

Sick leave, turnover and disruption alone account for $104.1 million dollars and initial treatment, probably in insurance payments totals $238.6 million. (Eddy, 1981, Page and Asire, 1985)

FOLLOW-UP

It has been well documented that the most valuable facet of cancer screening is regular follow-up. The Pennzoil Cancer Awareness Program has incorporated a comprehensive follow-up.

First, all new employees have the opportunity to be screened on a yearly basis. All employees found to be at risk for colon cancer will annually be sent a hemoccult slide kit and an abridged questionnaire to update our Cancer Prevention Center records. Should the employees, at any time during the year, develop abnormalities or symptoms, they will be scheduled to see the nurse specialist, and as necessary, a physician.

For all the women designated at some risk for breast cancer, a yearly recall system has also been developed. Women under 40 years of age should have an examination with the nurse specialist and a consultation to update our records. Women 40-50 years of age should also have a consultation with the nurse and a mammogram every two years. Women over 50 should have a yearly mammogram with their nurse's examination and consultation. Again, if the woman develops any symptoms or abnormalities in the interim, she is urged to call immediately, to schedule an appointment with the nurse specialist, who can examine her to assess the problem, and refer her to the appropriate follow-up.

CHANGES AND REVISIONS IN THE PROGRAM

The changes made in the Cancer Awareness Program were by and large, to simplify the program in terms of office management. The quality of the screening and lecture program was not to be compromised, only enhanced. By simplifying it, we did enhance it.

Lecture Presentation

As Davison has shown, physicians can most effectively persuade the public in terms of health care. (Davison, 1974) Although it is impressive to have physicians lecture, their time is very expensive.

Lecture and audience results can be effective having instead a Nurse Practitioner, Epidemiologist, or other well-versed staff member present cancer information lectures.

Risk Assessment Form and Scheduling

Instead of the American Cancer Society Risk Assessment Form, which was too complex for certain audiences, we developed our own one page, self-scoring risk form. The employee completed it while he/she sat in the audience. This eliminated the need for personalized letters on risk assessments and allowed the employee immediate feedback as to his/her potential risk.

If the individual at risk wants a consult with the nurse specialist, he/she schedules a consultation as he/she leaves the lecture room.

At that time, the individual is given:

1. an appointment card,
2. a long questionnaire,
3. consent forms to fill out and sign,
4. brochures explaining the Cancer Prevention Center,
5. and a hemoccult slide.

This reduces mailing cost, the possibility of the packet being lost in the mail, and allows for on-the-spot questions, directions and answers.

Reporting Results

Instead of a letter to the individual, the Nurse Screener indicates results at the close of the consultation and makes specific recommendations. Following mammograms, patients are told to call back and get results 2 days after the exam. Patients are given the results of their colonoscopic exam immediately following the exam.

When they call, if the report was negative (clear) a Nurse or Secretary can give the results; if positive (not good) a Nurse or physician relays the results.

The employee's personal physician and the employee both receive a one page assessment reporting findings and recommendations.

New ideas and suggestions are readily incorporated into the program or paper work, to enhance our efficacy and efficiency whenever possible.

PROGRAM EXPANSION

Pennzoil has already expanded the Cancer Awareness Program from the Houston Headquarters office to surrounding plants and offices in the district, including the offshore drilling and production rigs in the Gulf of Mexico.

The Program has also been taken to rigs, and production plants throughout the states of Louisiana and Mississippi. Plans are being made to take the Cancer Awareness Program to Colorado, California, Pennsylvania and New Mexico later this year and next year. Discussions have also concerned expanding the screening program to include skin cancer, particularly for the offshore rig workers.

The results of the screening from the rig and plant workers have not yet been tabulated. Since the demographics and environmental conditions are different from those at Pennzoil Place, some epidemiological differences are anticipated. The Cancer Prevention Center hopes to be able to make a positive impact on the Cancer Awareness of this population, much as it did at Pennzoil Headquarters.

The Kelsey-Seybold Foundation's Cancer Prevention Center has demonstrated that a comprehensive Cancer Awareness Program specifically designed for company employees can impact employee awareness and understanding of the disease. The success of the Pennzoil Cancer Awareness Program is indicative of the future promise for Cancer Education and Screening Programs in the workplace.

REFERENCES

Abercrombie, M.L.J., Ph.D. (1974): "Working with Groups," Health Education Theory and Practice in Cancer Control, UICC Technical Report Series, vol. 10: pgs. 28-33.

Clark, A.W., Ph.D. (1974): "Understanding and Changing Attitudes," Health Education Theory and Practice in Cancer Control, UICC Techical Report Series, vol. 10: pgs 69-80.

Cohen, William S. (Feb. 1985): "Health Promotion in the Workplace," American Psychologist, vol. 40, no. 2: pgs. 213-216.

Davison, R.L. (1974): "Special Considerations in Cancer Education Programmes," Health Education Theory and Practice in Cancer Control, UICC Technical Report Series, vol. 10: pgs. 64-68.

Development of Cancer Centres and Community Cancer Control Programmes Report on WHO Working Group, Luxembourg, 20-22 October 1981; WHO Regional Office for Europe, 1982: p. 10.

Duff, Jean F., M.A., M.P.H. (Sept. 1984): "Three Companies Encouraged by Results of Health Promotion," Occupational Health and Safety, vol. 53, no. 8: pgs. 82-86.

Eddy, D.M., "Guidelines for the Cancer-Related Check-Up: Recommendations and Rationale," CA-A Cancer Journal for Clinicians, 30: 194-240, 1980.

Eddy, D.M., "Economics of Cancer Prevention and Detection, Getting More for Less," Cancer, vol. 47, no. 5, March 1981.

James, Walter (1974); "Conduct of a Public
    Education Program," Health Education Theory
    and Practice in Cancer Control, UICC
    Technical Report Series, vol. 10: pgs. 21-27.

Mettlin, Curtis and Cummings, Michael, K.,
    (1983): "Experience with a Cancer Prevention-
    Detection Center," Cancer Prevention in
    Clinical Medicine, Raven Press, New York:
    pgs. 131-145.

Page, Harriet S., and Asire, Ardyce, J.,
    Cancer Rates and Risks, National Institutes
    of Health, no. 85-691, 1985, pp. 33-36.

Van Paris, L. G., and Eckhardt, S. (Sept 1984):
    Public Education in Primary and Secondary
    Cancer Prevention, In: Hygie, International
    Journal of Health Education, vol. 3: pgs.
    14-24.

RESEARCH ON CANCER CONTROL INTERVENTIONS

Advances in Cancer Control: The War on Cancer—
15 Years of Progress, pages 123–127
© 1987 Alan R. Liss, Inc.

IMPROVING CANCER PATIENTS' PAIN CONTROL THROUGH EDUCATION*

Barbara Rimer, Dr.P.H.
Michael Levy, M.D., Ph.D.
Martha K. Keintz, Sc.M.
Norma MacElwee, R.N.
Paul F. Engstrom, M.D.

The Fox Chase Cancer Center
Philadelphia, PA 19111

INTRODUCTION

The February 1986 issue of <u>Primary Care and Cancer</u>
contained a detailed case history of a 46 year old woman
whose unbearable lumbar pain was attributed to
adenocarcinoma of the rectum. Her physician prescribed
Percodan and Demerol but advised her to take as little as
possible. Not until Mrs. B. was referred to a pain clinic
at MD Anderson and put on around-the-clock treatment with
MS Contin[R] was her pain controlled (Hill 1986). This
illustrates a point that is sad but true. While at least
60% of cancer patients experience pain, much of this pain
remains poorly controlled (Bonica 1979). Lack of control
may be due to both patient and physician factors, including
misinformation about tolerance and addiction to narcotic
analgesics (Angell 1982; Jones et al 1984; Levy 1982; Rimer
et al in press).

We were challenged by the unsatisfactory state of
affairs to develop an educational intervention aimed at
improving cancer patients' pain control.

The overall study objectives are to:

1. Increase compliance with pain control regimens.

*Supported by grant PHS P50-CA34856, NCI DHHS.

2. Increase recognition and management of side effects of pain medicines.
3. Decrease misconceptions about tolerance and addiction to narcotic pain medications.

EVALUATION DESIGN

A randomized clinical trial with a Solomon Four-Group design is being used to assess the effectiveness of the intervention (Campbell, Stanley 1963). Figure 1 shows the evaluation design.

FIGURE 1

Evaluation Design

	Group	Pretest	Intervention	Posttest (4 weeks)
	A	X	X	X
R	B	X		X
	C		X	X
	D			X

Thus, patients in groups A and B receive pretests, groups A and C receive the intervention, and all patients are assigned to the posttest. The design permits an assessment of the effects of the intervention as well as of pretesting. The pretest is a brief (less than 10 minutes) interview conducted by an oncology nurse. The posttest also is brief but is conducted by telephone. The interview study variables include patient demographics, knowledge, concerns about tolerance and addiction, recall of drug information, compliance, perceived personal control, anxiety and satisfaction.

Eligible patients are those who (1) are being treated by a participating physician, (2) are 20 years of age or older, (3) have received a narcotic pain prescription for purposes other than post-surgical pain control, (4) have an expected survival of three months or more and (5) agree to be interviewed.

Eligible patients are identified by the oncology nurses who work in the outpatient medicine and radiation departments and the two off-campus physician practices. Interviews are conducted by an oncology nurse experienced in interviewing techniques.

EDUCATIONAL INTERVENTION

The intervention consists of both printed and interpersonal elements, including an initial counseling session with an oncology nurse, distribution of a wallet-sized card with the essential regimen information recorded, for example, name of medication and possible side effects, and provision of a booklet entitled, "No More Pain," which contains personalized information about the patient's pain control regimen. It is written simply (at a 5.8 grade level) and uses graphic images to reinforce the spoken word. The emphasis is on conveying specific action instructions and stimulating retention through the use of repetition and reinforcement (Rimer et al in press). The intervention elements were pretested extensively and found comprehensible to a diverse group of patients. Control group participants are offered the pain control booklet at the conclusion of the posttest interview to ensure the ethical treatment of all study subjects.

PRELIMINARY RESULTS

A total of 185 patients have now been entered into the study. Of the first 156 patients, 8% had breast cancers, 35% lung, 37% colorectal and 17% other sites. About 35% of the patients had regional metastases, 44% had distant metastases and 20% had none. For about 18% of participants, the study prescription was the first narcotic analgesic; for the remainder it represented a change of dose (11%), refill (49%) or change in medication (22%). The most common pain medicines were Dilaudid and Percocet. Patients were divided nearly evenly between men (52%) and women (48%). The mean age was 62 years. About 50% of respondents had less than a high school education. The majority were married (69%) or widowed (19%). Only one patient refused to complete the posttest; 13 patients were unable to complete it because they were incapacitated or had died.

A variety of methods were used for statistical

analysis, including Chi-square tests, t-tests,
Kruskal-Wallis and Wilcoxon tests, depending on the nature
of the variables.

There were no significant differences between the
experimental and control groups on any of the key study
variables at the pretest. Between the pretest and
posttest, there was a significant decrease in pain (p = .01)
for the experimental but not for the control group. There
was a trend toward a greater feeling of control over pain
in the experimental group (p = .15). There was a
significant difference between the study groups at the
posttest, with more of the experimental subjects taking the
correct dosage and more of the control group taking the
incorrect dosage of their pain medications (p = .02).
Also, significantly more of the experimental group recalled
being told something about how to take their pain
medication (p = .02). They were also more likely to have
done something to prevent the side effects of their pain
medications (p = .02).

The experimental group was less concerned that others
were worried about their possible addiction to pain
medication (p = .11) or that the medication would become
less effective in time (p = .005). Likewise, they were
less worried that others were concerned about tolerance
(p = .11). Lessening patient and family concerns about
tolerance and addiction were major foci of the
intervention.

There were some gender and education differences in
response to pain and perceptions about addiction and
tolerance within the experimental group. For example,
women reported more pain (p = .03) and were more worried
about addiction (p = .01). Younger (less than 60 years)
patients were more concerned about tolerance. Patients
with less than a high school education were significantly
more anxious than those with more than a high school
education (p = .04).

SUMMARY

While patient accrual for this study is not yet
complete, it appears that the intervention may be helping
patients to feel more in control over their pain, take the

correct medication dosage and take action to prevent side effects. At this point, the experimental subjects seem much less worried about tolerance to pain medications. The early results suggest some sociodemographic differences in response to pain which, if they persist, should probably be considered as factors in designing patient education programs.

REFERENCES

Angell M (1982). Quality of mercy. N Engl J Med 306:98-99.
Bonica J (1979). Importance of the problem. In Bonica J, Ventrafredd V (eds): "Advances in Pain Research and Therapy," New York: Raven Press, pp 1-12.
Campbell DT, Stanley JC (1963). "Experimental and Quasi-Experimental Designs for Research." Chicago: Rand McNally, pp 1-84.
Hill CS (1986). Patients in pain. Primary Care & Cancer 38-43.
Jones WL, Rimer B, Levy MH, Kinman JL (1984). Cancer patients' knowledge, beliefs, and behavior regarding pain control regimens: Implications for education programs. Pt Ed and Coun 5:159-164.
Levy M (1982). Clinical care of the terminal cancer patient. In Cassileth B, Cassileth P (eds): "Symptom Control Manual," Philadelphia: Lea and Febiger, pp 214-262.
Rimer B, Keintz MK, Levy M, Engstrom PF, Rodzwic D (in press). Cancer pain management: A clinical trial of an education program for patients. In "Advances in Cancer Control III: Health Care Financing and Research," New York: Alan R. Liss.

Advances in Cancer Control: The War on Cancer—
15 Years of Progress, pages 129–134
© 1987 Alan R. Liss, Inc.

A SURVEY OF CURRENT HEALTH SCREENING PRACTICES FOR
CHEMOTHERAPY HANDLERS

Linda Kratcha-Sveningson, R.N., M.S.;
Linda V. O'Halloran, R.N., M.S.

Community Clinical Oncology Program
St. Luke's Hospitals/Fargo Clinic
Fargo, North Dakota 58122

INTRODUCTION

In September 1983, St. Luke's Hospitals/Fargo Clinic
was the recipient of a Community Clinical Oncology Program
Grant from the National Cancer Institute. An integral
part of the St. Luke's CCOP is an outreach education and
consultation program for physicians and nurses practicing
in small community hospitals and clinics in our region.

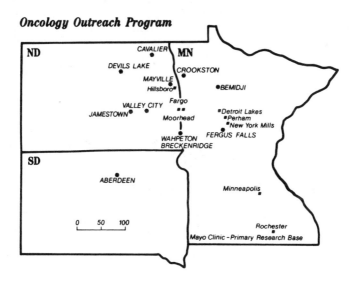

A major focus of nursing consultation to the CCOP affiliate clinics and hospitals has been the implementation of safe chemotherapy handling and administration practices. CCOP nurse consultants have assisted the clinics and hospitals in writing and instituting policies and procedures for the safe handling of cytotoxic agents.

Questions regarding actual risks to employees who handle chemotherapy agents was a frequent point of discussion during consultation visits. Additional questions were also asked: "Should there be health screening for chemotherapy handlers?" "If so, what is necessary and economially feasible and how often should health screens be conducted?"

Many studies have attempted to assess the occupational risk associated with the routine handling of chemotherapy agents (Falck 1979; Norppa 1980; Wasksvik 1981; Nikula 1984). These studies reported significant urine mutagenicity or chromosome abberrations in the blood of chemotherapy handlers. In contrast, other studies have found no evidence of mutagenic changes as a result of handling chemotherapy (Staino et al., 1981; Hoffman 1983; Gibson et al., 1984) Several reports by researchers have found evidence of biological absorption of cytotoxic drugs in chemotherapy handlers (Hirst et al., 1984; Jagun et al., 1982) taking minimal or no precautions during handling.

Guidelines for the safe handling of chemotherapy agents have been developed by many agencies and professional organizations (NIH 1982; Oncology Nursing Society 1984; American Society of Hospital Pharmacists 1983; OSHA 1986). However, recommendations for health screening of chemotherapy handlers are not clearly defined. The National Study Commission on Cytotoxic Exposure (March 1984) clearly states their recommendation:

"Certainly, it is a good idea to have routine examinations, but no specific 'markers' can be used now to monitor the effects of exposure to cytotoxic agents".

METHODOLOGY

In efforts to define the current standard of practice

in community hospitals for monitoring of cytotoxic exposure
among chemotherapy handlers, a questionnaire was designed
and sent to 64 randomly selected institutions from the
1983-84 ACCC membership roster and 12 member institutions
of the North Central Cancer Treatment Group.

RESULTS

Response to the survey was excellent with 60 of 76
(79% return rate) questionnaires returned within one month.
Fifty percent of the participating hospitals reported a
bed capacity of 301-600. As national trends have indicated,
respondents reported the administration of more chemotherapy
monthly in an outpatient setting than in a inpatient setting.
Fifty-three percent (32/60) of the respondents reported
that chemotherapy was administered by a designated chemotherapy nurse. The demographic data did not provide specific
indicators to predict the existence of health screening
practices in the participating institutions. Forty-four
of the sixty (73%) respondents reported that their chemotherapy handlers did not receive a periodic health screen
for purposes of monitoring cytotoxic exposure. Sixteen of
the sixty (27%) reported some form of health screen for
their chemotherapy handlers. Within this group, there was
much variation in what was included in the health screen.
The following were reported as components of the health
screen:

TABLE 1

Components of Health Screen	Incidence	
Complete Blood Count	13/16	81%
Platelet Count	6/16	38%
Urinalysis	8/16	50%
Chest X-Ray	4/16	25%
Blood Chemistry	4/16	25%
Electrocardiogram	1/16	6%
Liver/Kidney Function	1/15	6%
Assessment of Side Effects	3/15	19%

N - 16 Represents respondents conducting health screening

Ten of the sixteen (63%) participating institutions conducted yearly health screens; three (19%) conduct the screen every six months; and three (19%) institutions do C.B.C. and platelet count every three months.

DISCUSSION

This survey indicated that 73% of the participants reported no specific health examination for the purpose of assessing and monitoring the effects of cytotoxic exposure in chemotherapy handlers. The findings of this survey can not be generalized to all cancer care institutions as university hospitals and/or comprehensive cancer care centers were not surveyed. In retrospect, additional survey information that may have been benefical include the following:

1. Additional information from the institutions utilizing a health screen:

    a. How many handlers must be screened?

    b. What plan does the institution have for dealing with the individuals who have abnormal health screening findings?

    c. How are abnormal findings utilized to reduce future risk for fellow employees?

2. What precautions are utilized by chemotherapy handlers?

3. Are chemotherapy handlers logged for future reference or study?

As cancer care providers, we must continue to address our responsibility to chemotherapy handlers. Future endeavors must be directed at the following issues:

1. The efficacy of utilizing established chemotherapy handling guidelines as optimal protection for the chemotherapy handler.

2. The development of quality assurance programs that periodically evaluate and verify safe chemotherapy handling practices.

3.   Standardization of health screening for monitoring the effect of chemotherapy exposure.

4.   Continued research to identify "sensitive markers" that measure the effects of exposure to cytotoxic agents.

5.   Epidemiological studies to provide information of potential long term effects from cytotoxic exposure.

To summarize, this survey depicts variation in practice for the monitoring of cytotoxic exposure in chemotherapy handlers among community hospitals and clinics. The literature recommends a routine examination for chemotherapy handlers but provides limited and inclusive data for what specific studies will measure the effects of cytotoxic exposure. Therefore, it is imperative that oncology nurses continue to question their potential risk as chemotherapy handlers and continue to support research endeavors that may answer these questions.

This investigation was supported by PHS Grant CA 37417 awarded by the National Cancer Institute.

REFERENCES

American Society of Hospital Pharmacists (1983). Procedure for handling cytotoxic drugs.

Falck K, Grohn P, Sorsa M, Vainio H, Heinonen E, Holsti L. (1979) Mutagenicity in urine of nurses handling cytostatic drugs. Lancet 1:1250-1251.

Gibson JF, Gompertz D, Hedworth-Whitty RB (1984). Mutagenicity of urine from nurses handling cytotoxic drugs. Lancet 11:100-101.

Hirst M, Mills DG, Tse S, Levin L (1984). Occupational exposure to cyclophosphamide. Lancet 1:186-8.

Hoffman D (1983). Lack of urine mutagenicity of nurses administering pharmacy prepared doses of antineoplastic agents. American Journal of Intravenous Therapy 10:28-30.

Jagun O, Ryan M, Waldron HA (1982). Urinary thioether excretion in nurses handling cytotoxic drugs. Lancet 2:443-4.

National Institutes of Health (1982). Recommendations for the safe handling of parenteral antineoplastic drugs.

National Study Commission on Cytotoxic Exposure (1984). Consensus responses to unresolved questions concerning cytotoxic agents.

Neal A, Wadden RA, Chou WL (1983). Exposure of hospital workers to airborne antineoplastic agents. American Journal of Hospital Pharmacy 40:597-601.

Nikula E, Kivinitty K, Leisti S, et al (1984). Chromosome aberrations in lymphocytes of nurses handling cytostatic drugs. Scandiavian Journal Work Environmental Health 10:71-74.

Norppa H, Sorea M, Vainio H, et al (1980). Increased sister chromatid exchange in lymphocytes of nurses handling cytostatic drugs. Scandiavian Journal of Work Environmental Health 6:299-301.

Oncology Nursing Society (1984). Cancer chemotherapy: guidelines and recommendations for nursing education and practice.

Staino N, Galleli JF, Adamson RH, Thorgierson SS (1981). Lack of mutagenic activity in urine from hospital pharmacists admixing antitumor drugs. Lancet 2:615-616.

United States Department of Labor. Occupational Safety and Health Administration (1986). Guidelines for cytotoxic (antineoplastic) drugs.

Waksvic H, Brogger A, Klepp O (1981). Chromosome analyses of nurses handling cytostatic drugs. Cancer Treatment Reports 65:607-610.

Advances in Cancer Control: The War on Cancer—
15 Years of Progress, pages 135–144
© 1987 Alan R. Liss, Inc.

PROCESS AND IMPACT EVALUATION OF A CANCER PROGRAM FOR OLDER PEOPLE*

Linda Fleisher, M.P.H.
Barbara Rimer, Dr.P.H.
Martha K. Keintz, Sc.M.
Paul F. Engstrom, M.D.
Christine Wilson, M.A.

The Fox Chase Cancer Center
Philadelphia, PA   19111

BACKGROUND

Cancer is disproportionately widespread among older adults, with 55% of cancers occurring in persons 65 and older (Peterson et al 1979; Yancik 1983). In addition, the elderly harbor misconceptions about cancer and may wait longer to report symptoms than younger people (Kegeles, Grady 1982; Rimer et al 1983). Age is an important risk factor for cancer, and educating the older person about the efficacy of screening and detection is crucial.

The "Cancer Education Program for Older Citizens" (CAPROC) is a randomized community study whose goal is to assess whether older people exposed to a tailored cancer education program are more likely than unexposed older people to: (a) increase their knowledge about cancer, (b) strengthen their beliefs in the efficacy of cancer screening tests and early detection, (c) strengthen their intentions to take appropriate action in the face of cancer warning signs, (d) discuss recommended cancer screening tests with their physicians and have the tests and (e) take appropriate action if they have experienced potential cancer symptoms.

Ideally, comprehensive evaluation includes three

*Supported by grant PHS P50-CA34856, NCI DHHS.

levels--process, impact and outcome (Donabedian 1973; Green et al 1980; Green, Lewis 1986). Process evaluation documents what is actually happening on a day-to-day basis, and provides information about the participants' satisfaction with the program (Green et al 1980; Patton 1978; Rimer et al in press; Suchman 1967; Weiss 1972; Windsor et al 1984).

Impact evaluation measures knowledge, attitudes, behavioral intentions and behaviors and assesses the immediate and intermediate effects of a program. Outcome evaluation measures the changes in morbidity, mortality and quality of life (Green et al 1980; Green, Lewis 1986).

This paper will focus on the study results from the second of two target communities, the Kensington area of Philadelphia.

STUDY QUESTIONS

The following research questions will be addressed:

1. Was participation in the follow-up interview influenced by program implementation factors, such as group size or logistical problems?
2. Was participant satisfaction with the program influenced by program implementation?
3. Were there changes in the beliefs, attitudes, knowledge, behavioral intentions and behaviors of the participants?
4. Were the impact changes influenced by program implementation or participant satisfaction?

METHODS

Between September 1984 and June 1985, over 1400 (n = 1406) older people meeting in 21 church clubs received either the experimental cancer education program, "Help Yourself to Health," or a control program about physical fitness called, "Getting Fitter Every Day." The cancer program had three components: (a) an audiovisual presentation designed to reduce false beliefs and increase knowledge about cancer and to improve communication between the elderly and their physicians about cancer, (b) group discussion led by an oncology nurse and (c) a booklet that reviewed gender-specific cancer screening tests recommended for men and women over the age of 50. Some respondents also received a fourth intervention, telephone counseling from an oncology nurse. The fitness program consisted of three components analogous to those used for the cancer program.

The programs were designed to be both informative and entertaining. The presentations and educational materials relied extensively on repetition and reinforcement. In addition, all materials were found to be comprehensible to persons with an 8th grade reading level.

We employed a randomized pretest-posttest design in which all the senior groups associated with churches in the defined geographic area were assigned randomly to receive the experimental or control program and then to receive a pretest or only an abbreviated set of demographic questions. Telephone posttest interviews were conducted by professional interviewers with consenting participants at six weeks and six months after the program.

Qualitative and quantitative process data were collected at two points. First, during the programs, a staff member completed an observational checklist, which included items such as estimated size of the audience and logistical problems, and recorded comments and questions of participants. Second, during the sixth-week interview, participant satisfaction was measured using a four-item scale of program attributes: informative, useful, encouraging and upsetting.

Impact items were collected at all three data collection points and assessed knowledge, beliefs, attitudes and behavioral intentions using Likert-type items generating a four-point ordinal scale. Health behaviors were measured using a dichotomous response. For example, "In the last month did you have a bowel exam?"

TARGET POPULATION

The Kensington area is a predominately white community, occupationally blue-collar and working class. The housing units are primarily row homes, and

residential areas are mixed with industrial tracts. It is
a stable, traditional neighborhood.

The socio-demographic characteristics of the
respondents by type of program are summarized in Table 1.
The respondents were predominately female (82%), and over
three-fourths of the participants were between the ages of
60 and 75 (79%). Only 24% of the participants in the
Kensington community had graduated high school. In fact,
39% had 8 years or less of schooling.

ACCRUAL

We requested permission for further follow-up with the
participants after the pretest. The overall permission
rate for the Kensington community was 64%. This permission
rate was not as high as the first community, Fox Chase,
which was 72%. However, the Kensington community is very
close-knit and somewhat suspicious of outsiders. Once
participants entered the study, their retention rate was
quite high. The completion rate of the sixth-week posttest
was 71%; 97% of those completing the sixth-week interview
gave permission for follow-up, and sixth-month interviews
were completed with 92% of them.

Denomination was the socio-demographic variable most
closely related to permission for follow-up. Catholic
groups had lower permission rates. It is difficult to say
whether this is truly a denominational difference. It may
reflect the purpose of the Catholic groups which tended to
be more socially and recreationally oriented.

RESULTS

The first study question refers to one of the most
important functions of the process analysis, which is to
determine the relationship between program implementation
and permission for follow-up.

We found that, as group size increased, permission
rates declined. This effect was most profound for groups
over 200 people. Permission rates were significantly lower
in groups where there were two or more logistical problems,
such as starting late or problems administering the

TABLE 1

**SOCIO-DEMOGRAPHIC CHARACTERISTICS OF PARTICIPANTS
WHO COMPLETED PRETEST BY PROGRAM TYPE**

(n = 1406)

Characteristics	Experimental		Control	
	n	(%)	n	(%)
Gender				
Male	120	(20)	132	(16)
Female	485	(80)	669	(84)
Age*				
60–75	497	(82)	612	(76)
$\geq$ 76	108	(18)	189	(24)
Education				
< 8 years	223	(38)	317	(40)
9–11 years	215	(36)	299	(38)
H.S. graduate	116	(20)	124	(16)
> H.S.	39	(6)	45	(6)
Marital Status*				
Married	284	(47)	312	(39)
Widowed	276	(46)	412	(52)
Never married or other	42	(7)	75	(9)
Perceived Health Status				
Better	232	(39)	294	(37)
About the same	333	(56)	434	(56)
Worse	29	(5)	53	(7)

*$p \leq .01$, using Chi-Square Statistic

pretest, and significantly higher (p < .01) for those groups where more than 10 questions were asked. Women were most affected by the implementation variables. Permission rates for women were significantly higher in small groups (p < .001), lower in groups over 200 (p < .001) and where there were two or more problems. These trends were confirmed for other demographic variables, such as age and education. For example, participants between the ages of 60 and 75 were significantly more likely to give permission for follow-up (p = .02).

The program was rated highly by participants, with a mean satisfaction score of 17.8 out of 20. Table 2 shows participant satisfaction by program type and selected demographic variables. The only significant differences in participant satisfaction were on the attributes "upsetting" and "useful;" while still finding the program not very upsetting, the cancer program participants found the program more upsetting than the fitness participants. Protestant participants rated the program significantly higher than the Catholics on all four attributes.

We found considerable interaction between the program implementation variables and participant satisfaction. As group size increased, participants of both programs rated the program less useful, encouraging and were generally less satisfied. In the cancer group, as more questions were asked, the ratings on all four attributes and total satisfaction increased.

The third study question addresses the impact of the program. Here, we consider representative items from four categories: knowledge, efficacy, behavioral intention and self-reported health behaviors. Table 3 summarizes these findings.

Knowledge. The core factual message of the cancer program is the relationship between age and cancer risk. At the pretest, the overwhelming majority of participants disagreed that "older people are more likely to get cancer than younger people." At both the sixth-week (p < .01) and sixth-month (p < .05) posttests, the experimental group was significantly more likely to recognize that age is related to cancer risk.

Efficacy. At both the sixth-week (p = .03) and

TABLE 2

PARTICIPANT SATISFACTION RESPONSES FROM SIXTH-WEEK POSTTEST
BY PROGRAM TYPE AND SELECTED DEMOGRAPHIC VARIABLES

Kensington Community

Kruskal-Wallis One-Way Analysis of Variance

	Program Type	Age	Gender	Denomination
How _____ was the program?				
Informative				.00
Useful	.00			.00
Encouraging			.03	.00
Upsetting	.00			.02
Total Satisfaction Score		.03	.04	.00

$p \leq .05$

TABLE 3

PERCENT GIVING THE MOST DESIRED RESPONSE TO PROGRAM IMPACT VARIABLES ON THE SIXTH-WEEK AND SIXTH-MONTH POSTTESTS BY PROGRAM TYPE

Kensington Community

Impact Variables	Sixth-Week Posttest (n = 638)		Sixth-Month Posttest (n = 569)	
	Experimental	Control	Experimental	Control
[a] Knowledge				
• Age as a cancer risk factor	32 ***	20	32 ***	20
[a] Efficacy				
• Cancer screening tests	73 ***	62	67 **	57
• Early detection	73	67	64	59
• Treatments	35	27	25 ***	18
[a] Behavioral Intention				
• Change in a mole	89	90	89	89
• Persistent indigestion	82	86	85	81
• Hoarse voice	88 ***	77	90 ***	81
[b] Behavior				
• Bowel examination	22	22	34	30
• Skin examination	24	20	44 **	34
• Breast examination	--	--	50 ***	35
• Breast self-examination	67	65	73	68
• Asked about cancer tests	14	12	23 ***	11

* p < .10   ** p < .06   *** p < .01

[a] Kruskal-Wallis One-Way Analysis of Variance, using a four-point ordinal scale
[b] Chi-Square Contingency Table, using a dichotomous response

sixth-month (p = .02) posttests, cancer participants were significantly more likely to believe in the efficacy of cancer screening tests. At six months, cancer participants also showed a significant differential belief in the efficacy of cancer treatments (p = .002).

Behavioral Intention. On the sixth-week posttest, cancer group participants (p = .01) showed a significantly greater intention to seek medical advice for a hoarse voice. This positive change in behavioral intention was maintained at the sixth-month posttest.

Behaviors. There were significant differences between the study groups in their health behaviors. At the sixth-month posttest, cancer group participants were more likely to have had a skin examination (p = .02), to have asked their doctors questions about cancer tests (p = .001) and to have had a breast examination (p = .001).

The last study question addresses the relationship between process and impact measures.

The finding of most relevance for program planning was the strong relationship between finding the program upsetting and the reduced likelihood of having had a bowel (p = .02), skin (p = .001) and breast examination (p = .02) or to have asked their doctor about cancer screening tests (p = .02). This is consistent with past health education research that shows too high a level of fear arousal can be counterproductive (Leventhal et al 1965).

DISCUSSION

The results suggest that much can be learned from collecting both process and impact data. The clear interrelationsiip between program implementation and permission for follow-up is of special relevance to professionals conducting research with older adults. It appears that a group of less than 100 older adults is optimal for obtaining high follow-up rates.

The impact evaluation shows that the program was successful in improving knowledge about cancer risk, belief in the efficacy of cancer tests and early detection. It also shows that older people who are exposed to a tailored cancer education program are more likely to seek medical advice for some of the cancer warning signs and to practice some of the recommended screening behaviors.

REFERENCES

Donabedian A (1973). "Aspects of Medical Care Administration." Cambridge: Harvard University Press.
Green LW, Kreuter MW, Deeds SG, Partridge KD (1980). "Health Education Planning: A Diagnostic Approach." Palo Alto: Mayfield, pp 134-136.
Green LW, Lewis FM (1986). "Measurement and Evaluation in Health Education and Health Promotion." Palo Alto: Mayfield, pp 27-52.
Kegeles S, Grady K (1982). Behavioral dimensions. In Schottenfeld D, Fraumeni J (eds): "Cancer Epidemiology and Prevention," Philadelphia: Saunders, pp 1049.
Leventhal H, Jones S, Singer R (1965). Effects of fear and specificity of recommendation upon attitudes and behaviors. Journal of Personality and Social Psychology 2:20-29.
Patton MQ (1978). "Utilization-Focused Evaluation." Beverly Hills: Sage, pp 149-177.
Peterson BH, Kennedy BJ, Butler RN, Gastel B (1979). Aging and cancer management. CA-A Cancer Journal for Clinicians 29:322-340.
Rimer B, Jones WL, Wilson C, Bennett D, Engstrom PF (1983). Planning a cancer control program for older citizens. The Gerontologist 23:384-389.
Rimer B, Keintz M, Glassman B, Kinman J (in press). Health education for older persons: Lessons from research and program evaluations. Annual Review of Health Education.
Suchman EA (1967). "Evaluation Research: Principles and Practice in Public Service and Social Action Program." New York: Russell Sage, pp 66-68.
Weiss CH (1972). "Evaluation Research." Englewood Cliffs: Prentice-Hall.
Windsor RA, Baranowski T, Clark N, Cutter G (1984). "Evaluation of Health Promotion and Education Programs." Palo Alto: Mayfield, pp 88-125.
Yancik R (1983). Frame of reference: Old age as the context for the prevention and treatment of cancer. In Yancik R (ed): "Perspectives on Prevention and Treatment of Cancer in the Elderly," New York: Raven Press, pp 5-17.

Advances in Cancer Control: The War on Cancer—
15 Years of Progress, pages 145-152
© 1987 Alan R. Liss, Inc.

FREE BREAST CANCER SCREENING UTILIZATION AND RESULTS

Sharon W. Davis, M.P.A.
Christine M. Wilson, M.A.
Paul F. Engstrom, M.D.
Bienvenido T. Samson, M.D.

Fox Chase Cancer Center
Philadelphia, PA   19111

INTRODUCTION

Breast cancer screening can save lives. Yet only 15 percent of U.S. women over 50 have a mammogram every year (King, 1985). In order to encourage eligible women, the Fox Chase Cancer Center offered free mammography and breast examinations performed by a physician. In this paper, I will briefly discuss the rationale behind mammography and complimentary physical examinations as breast cancer screening techniques. Then I will describe the free breast cancer screening program offered by the Fox Chase Cancer Center and the results we obtained.

Concept Behind Early Detection

Studies of large numbers of women screened by mammography have shown significant reductions in breast cancer mortality (see Table 1). For example, the Health Insurance Plan trial conducted in New York in the 1960's showed that women offered screening by mammography and physical exam had a one-third reduction in mortality from breast cancer. Reduced mortality is still evident on 10-14 year follow-up (Feig, 1984). A later study in the Netherlands suggested a 50-70% reduction of breast cancer deaths in women who were screened by mammography (Harvard, 1984). Similarly, a randomized trial started in Sweden in 1977 showed an overall reduction in mortality of 31 percent for women receiving regular breast cancer screening (Tabar, et al, 1985).

TABLE 1

REDUCTION OF BREAST CANCER DEATHS
FOR WOMEN SCREENED BY MAMMOGRAPHY

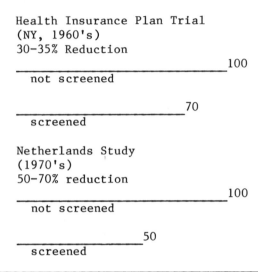

Health Insurance Plan Trial
(NY, 1960's)
30-35% Reduction
_____ 100
    not screened

_____ 70
    screened

Netherlands Study
(1970's)
50-70% reduction
_____ 100
    not screened

_____ 50
    screened

Breast cancer screening reduces mortality by detecting breast cancers early, even before they are palpable, when the chances for cure are the highest (see Table 2). Studies have found ten year survival rates of 80 to 90 percent for women with early breast cancer (defined as a mass of 2 centimeters in diameter or less, with no involvement of the lymph nodes). Survival rates drop down to 40% for women with 2-5 centimeter breast cancers and with involved nodes (Council Report, 1984).

TABLE 2

TEN-YEAR SURVIVAL, BY STAGE, OF PATIENTS WITH BREAST CANCER

Stage (Pathologic)	Tumor Size, cm	Nodes	Approximate Ten-Year Survival, %
I	<1	no	90
I	1-2	no	80
II	2-5	no	70
		yes	40
III	>5	yes	10-20
IV	Distant metasteses		Rare

Mammography and Physical Examination as Methods

Mammography is the most effective screening technique to detect early breast cancer. However, mammographic study of the breast should be conducted in conjunction with a physical examination performed by a well-trained individual. Mammography and physical examination together accounted for the largest percentage of breast cancers detected in the recent Breast Cancer Detection Demonstration Projects (American Cancer Society, 1982).

THE FOX CHASE PROGRAM

Process for Application and Exams

The Fox Chase Cancer Center offered free mammography and breast cancer screening examinations performed by a physician. The program was advertised in 14 local weekly newspapers during breast awareness week in October, 1985. The advertisements focused on the positive actions that women could take with the headline "Women Over 35 - A Breast Exam Could Save Your Life."

Respondents were encouraged to complete a risk assessment included in the advertisement and return it to the Center within a month. Based on the information included in the risk assessments, women were placed into three risk categories: 1) symptomatic (women who indicated any of the breast cancer symptoms), 2) women needing a breast examination (any non-symptomatic woman over 35 who had not had a recent mammogram), and 3) women who were not eligible for an exam at the time (women under age 35, or those who had received a mammogram within the past year).

Two-hundred and sixty-four women returned risk assessments during the study period (see Table 3). Eighty-two of these women indicated breast symptoms, about one-third of the total. Women without symptoms who were eligible for examinations made up the largest group, with 169 women representing 64 percent of the total risk assessments. There were only 13 women who were not eligible for the examination, or just under 5 percent. All women returning risk assessments received a letter corresponding to their risk category.

TABLE 3

RISK CATEGORIES

Category	Number	Percentage
symptomatic	82	31.1
need exam	169	64.0
no exam	13	4.9
	264	100.0

Mammograms and breast examinations were completed on two separate visits to allow the examining physician to use the mammography results. Both the women and their primary physicians received written reports on the results of their examinations. Women were allowed to chose where they would receive follow-up care.

Educational Materials

Several educational materials were included in the packet sent to women returning risk assessments, in addition to the letter corresponding to risk category. The National Cancer Institute booklet on breast examinations, the American Cancer Society guidelines on mammography, and a pamphlet on the Fox Chase Cancer Center Breast Evaluation Center were enclosed.

Results

The majority of eligible women followed through with scheduling an appointment and receiving both examinations (see Table 4). Of the 251 women who were eligible for the program, 193 (77%) called and scheduled an appointment for a mammogram. Fourteen women who had scheduled appointments did not show up for the mammogram, and an additional 14 women dropped out of the program after receiving a mammogram but before receiving a physical examination. Thus, 66 percent of eligible women completed the entire program.

TABLE 4

PROGRAM COMPLIANCE

Respondents	Number	Percentage
total respond.	264	100.0
not eligible	13	4.9
eligible	251	95.1

Compliance	Number	Percentage of Eligibles (251)
scheduled	193	77
mammogram	179	71
physical ex.	165	66

A surprisingly large proportion of women had abnormal mammograms (see Table 5). Twenty-six mammograms were interpreted as being abnormal, or 15 percent. An additional 26 mammograms showed fibrocystic disease with some abnormality. The majority of women, 54 percent, had fibrocystic breasts, but no abnormalities. Thirty mammograms were classified as negative, with no evidence of a fibrocystic condition.

Physical exam results were abnormal for 33 women, or 20 percent. Cross-tabulations demonstrate that mammograms and physical examinations are complimentary, since there was not an exact correlation between the two. Three women who had received a normal mammogram were found to have some abnormality upon physical examination.

Malignancies were suspected for 16 women, or 9 percent of eligible participants. The examining physician was asked to indicate, for the abnormal examinations, whether or not malignancy was suspected. For women who did not complete the physical examination, this was determined from the mammogram. Cross-tabulations indicate that symptoms were not a good predictor of malignancy. Nine of the women who reported no symptoms on the risk assessment had an abnormality which was suspected to be malignant.

TABLE 5

MAMMOGRAM RESULTS

Result	Number	Percentage
abnormal	26	15
FCD (ab)	26	15
FCD (norm)	97	54
normal	30	17
	179	100

PHYSICAL EXAM RESULTS		
Result	Number	Percentage
abnormal	33	20
normal	132	80
	165	100

SUSPECTED MALIGNANCIES: 16 (9%)

Non-routine follow-up care was recommended for 42 women, or 23 percent of the women receiving mammograms.

TABLE 6

FOLLOW-UP CARE RECOMMENDED

Type	Number	Percentage
Re-exam	12	28.6
Biopsy	16	38.1
Other	14	33.3
	42	100.0

Total follow-up (42) represents 23% of total 179 examinations

Re-examination within three months was recommended for 12 women, biopsy for 16 women, and other types of follow-up for

14 women. Other types of follow-up included ultrasound, comparison of previous mammograms, or monitoring of lumps by the patient. All women were instructed in breast self-examination, and were told when to obtain their next mammogram.

CONCLUSIONS

In conclusion, the free breast cancer screening offered at the Fox Chase Cancer Center was able to generate responses from appropriate risk categories of women. That the program attracted so many symptomatic women who were not receiving ongoing care from a physician is particularly revealing - the implication is that, even with an obvious breast cancer symptom, cost is a major factor for some women in preventing prompt screening and diagnosis. The high proportion of women (23%) from the study for whom non-routine follow-up was recommended demonstrates the success of the program in detecting breast problems. No definitive results are available yet on the actual number of breast cancers found because women were allowed to choose where they would obtain follow-up care. However, the number of suspected malignancies is quite high (9%).

TABLE 7

RATE OF SUSPECTED MALIGNANCY

Study	Number	Percent
Fox Chase	16	9
BCDD	--	4*

*biopsies performed

In comparison, biopsy rates per 10,000 women screening during the Breast Cancer Detection Demonstration Project were 358.1 for the first year, or almost 4 per 100 women (Baker, 1982). We must conclude that free breast examinations, made available to women without unnecessary difficulty, can be an important way to detect breast cancers early, and thus, to save lives.

REFERENCES

King, Martha   Autumn (1985).   "Mammography - Good News, Bad
News" Cancer News, American Cancer Society, Inc., p. 2.

Feig, Stephen A., M.D. (1984).   "Validity of Mammographic
Screening: Pros and Cons." Editorial, Cancer Investigation,
2(2), 177-179.

The Harvard Medical School Health Letter (1984).   Mammography
- New Data, Volume IX, Number 11.

Tabar, L., C.J.G. Fagerberg, A. Gad, L. Baldetorp, L.H.
Holmberg, O. Grontoft, U. Ljungquist, B. Lundstrom, J.C.
Manson (1985). "Reduction in Mortality form Breast Cancer
After Mass Screening with Mammography." The Lancet, Saturday
13 April, pp.829-832.

Council Report (1984), "Early Detection of Breast Cancer",
Council on Scientific Affairs, JAMA, Dec 7, Vol. 252, No. 21,
pp.3008-3011.

American Cancer Society, National Task Force on Breast Cancer
Control (1982). Cancer News, Autumn, pp.5-6.
Baker, Larry H., M.D.(1982). "Breast Cancer Detection
Demonstration Project: Five-Year Summary Report,"
Ca-A Cancer Journal for Clinicians. Vol. 32, No. 4.

Advances in Cancer Control: The War on Cancer—
15 Years of Progress, pages 153–160
© 1987 Alan R. Liss, Inc.

A CANCER PATIENT SURVEY TO HELP DETERMINE PSYCHOSOCIAL
NEEDS, DESIGN, AND IMPLEMENT MEANINGFUL INTERVENTIONS

Morry Edwards, M.A., Borgess Mental Health Center

Nancy White, R.N., M.S., Borgess Medical Center,
1521 Gull Road, Kalamazoo, Michigan 49001

INTRODUCTION

The Cancer Counseling Program (CCP), as a part of the
Borgess Medical Center Oncology Program, has been providing
supportive services to area cancer patients for over eight
years. The overall goal of the Cancer Counseling Program is
to provide the cancer patients and family with psycho-
logical support using both individual and group formats.
Much of the programming had been based more on staff perception of the patient needs rather than an actual assessment of patient desires. While there were a number of
advertised free psychosocial interventions such as a "drop-
in" discussion group and a stress management class,
attendance was often sporadic and poor though spirited. In
order to design and implement more meaningful interventions,
a brief, simple and anonymous survey was administered to
100 patients in our outpatient cancer clinic. The results
obtained were then used to remodel existing programs as
well as structure new services.

METHOD AND SUBJECT SAMPLE

Between September and December of 1985, a 14-item
questionnaire was administered to 100 cancer patients that
were receiving services in the outpatient clinic at Borgess
Medical Center (using an accidental sampling process). One
survey was discounted because the person did not have cancer
and was being treated at the clinic for a hematologic dis-
order. The questionnaires were handed to the patient when
he/she signed-in at the reception desk. The questionnaire

was then immediately completed and returned to the
receptionist. A non-significant number of people refused to
fill out the survey. Results were not tabulated until all
surveys were collected. Patients could sign their names if
they desired, otherwise they were not identified except for
four pieces of information: diagnosis, county of residence,
age and sex. The demographics of this subject sample are
presented in the following four tables.

Table 1

DIAGNOSIS

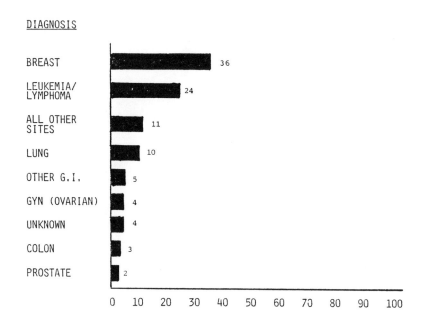

Table 2

COUNTY OF RESIDENCE

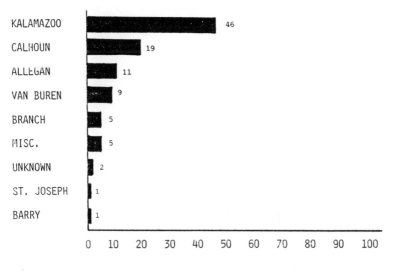

Table 3

AGE OF PARTICIPANTS

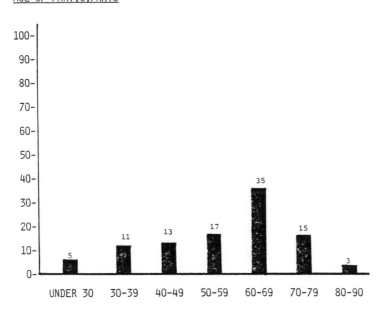

Table 4

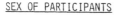

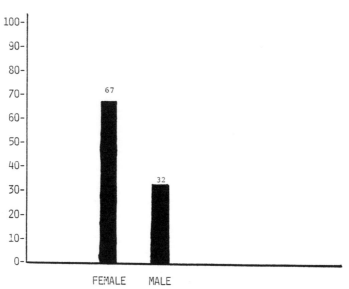

RESULTS

The responses are presented in the next ten tables (Table 5 through 14). The survey item is stated exactly as it appeared in the questionnaire. The left side of the table tabulates the response and is to be viewed vertically. The figure on the right side of the table represents the reason a respondent checked "no" and is to be viewed horizontally. Four of the survey items are not included since they covered areas such as meeting times for the groups and desire to work on the clinic newsletter.

Table 5

I WOULD LIKE SOMEONE TO TALK TO ME ABOUT WHAT SERVICES ARE AVAILABLE AT
BORGESS MEDICAL CENTER CANCER COUNSELING PROGRAM.

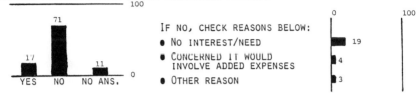

Table 6

I AM INTERESTED IN GETTING READING MATERIALS ABOUT CANCER AND RELATED
TOPICS.

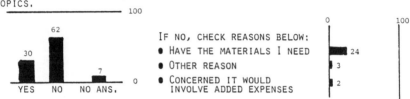

Table 7

I WOULD LIKE A CANCER COUNSELOR/NURSE/DOCTOR TO TALK TO ME ABOUT MY
DISEASE.

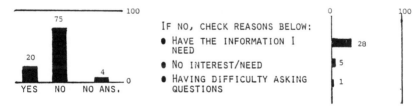

Table 8

I WOULD LIKE TO TALK TO A CANCER COUNSELOR.

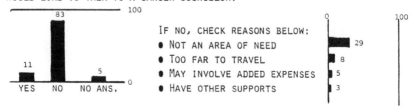

Table 9

I WOULD BE INTERESTED IN JOINING AN EDUCATIONAL/INFORMATIONAL GROUP WITH
OTHER CANCER PATIENTS.

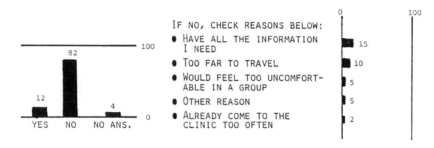

Table 10

I AM INTERESTED IN LEARNING HOW TO RELAX.

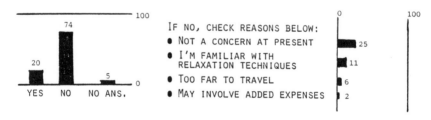

Table 11

I WOULD ATTEND A CLASS TO LEARN RELAXATION TECHNIQUES.

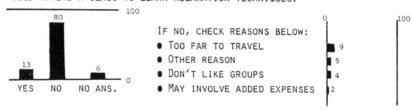

Table 12

I WOULD LIKE A CANCER COUNSELOR/NURSE/DOCTOR TO TALK TO FAMILY MEMBER(S) ABOUT CANCER.

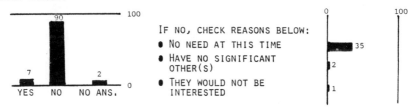

Table 13

I WOULD BE INTERESTED IN RECEIVING A NEWSLETTER ABOUT COPING WITH CANCER AND ITS TREATMENT.

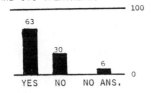

Table 14

I WOULD BE INTERESTED IN AN ONGOING SUPPORT GROUP FOR CANCER PATIENTS AND THEIR FAMILIES.

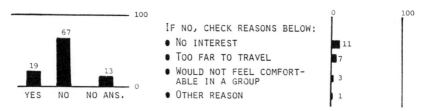

DISCUSSION AND CONCLUSIONS

The majority of patients appear to feel that they are knowledgeable about the support services available to them and they have no current desire or need for supportive services. The majority of patients also feel they neither need additional opportunities to talk to staff or a counselor nor have family members talk to the health care team. Since the majority of patients are also obtaining as much information as they feel they need, we are inferring that the staff is perceived as adequately accessible and responsive to their needs. A variable that may have influenced the respondents' answers, but was not determined, is the length of time from diagnosis.

Because several of our psychosocial support functions were poorly attended, the results of the survey enabled us to make several changes in our program. Because most of the patients perceived no need for an educational/informational or ongoing support group, our weekly unstructured "drop-in" group was radically modified. The format now features a specialized topic once a month with a professional speaker. The topics selected are those suggested by the patients or support persons. A five session stress management class that taught a variety of relaxation strategies and covered stressful concerns specific to cancer patients was offered five times yearly. Because the majority of patients did not feel a need to learn relaxation techniques and fewer stated they would want to attend a class, the stress management class will only be offered three times a year. Lastly, an extremely large percentage of those surveyed were interested in receiving a clinic newsletter. As a result, a bi-monthly newsletter has begun and more emphasis will be placed on it to meet informational and supportive needs in a way which is non-threatening and requires a minimum of patient time and energy.

Advances in Cancer Control: The War on Cancer—
15 Years of Progress, pages 161–172
© 1987 Alan R. Liss, Inc.

COMPARATIVE METHODOLOGIES FOR THE COMMUNITY DISTRIBUTION OF A
CANCER RISK ASSESSMENT FORM

Andrew M. Balshem, B.A.
Zili Amsel, Sc.D.
Doris Gillespie
Ann Guidera-Matey, M.S.
Paul Engstrom, M.D.

Fox Chase Cancer Center
Philadelphia, PA 19111

As part of our program in cancer control at the
Fox Chase Cancer Center we are developing a prototypic
community-based intervention program in an area of
Philadelphia experiencing higher than expected mortality from
cancer (Dayal et al, 1984). The program, which is modelled
on the basis of the North Karelia (Puska et al, 1983) and the
Stanford (Farquhar, 1978) cardiovascular disease programs, is
designed to heighten the awareness of community residents
about the risks of getting cancer and the ways they can
reduce these risks. The overall goal of our program is to
alter knowledge, attitudes and practices in order to have a
positive impact on morbidity and mortality due to cancer.
Short term goals include:

(1) modifying the image held by community residents of
    cancer, cancer treatments, and treatment outcomes;
(2) promoting early treatment by encouraging the prac-
    tice of self-surveillance and the use of local
    screening facilities;
(3) reducing cancer risks by modifying personal habits.

There are five principal components to our project:

(1) a community awareness campaign to educate and inform
    the public about cancer and what our program offers;

Supported by NCI-PHS Grant #CA34856.

(2) a self-administered, site-specific cancer risk
    assessment form;
(3) a screening program designed to familiarize resi-
    dents with cancer detection procedures and to
    identify early stage cancers;
(4) health education programs (for children and adults)
    to modify health beliefs, alter smoking patterns,
    and increase nutritional awareness;
(5) individual health counseling.

The focus of this paper is the self-administered risk
assessment form. The form has the potential to serve two
purposes for this project: as an epidemiologic tool, to
establish point prevelance rates of cancer risk in a defined
population, and as an intervention device, to raise the level
of awareness of one's risk for getting cancer in order to
motivate individuals to participate in screening and
detection and associated counseling services. Presented in
this paper are the results of a methodological study to
assess the best method for distribution of a cancer risk
assessment form. For this paper, the criteria for "best
method" is that method yielding the highest return rate.
Future analyses will address issues of representativeness or
internal validity. The methods of distribution that were
used in this analysis include:

(1) mail distribution (to neighborhoods characterized as
    having "strong" or "weak" support for our program);
(2) person to person at a "community pride" fair;
(3) person to person at a program-sponsored parade;
(4) person to person, following Mass, at local
    churches.

BACKGROUND

In our review of the literature we sought to find
information about risk assessment forms with a comparable
intent to our own. This review focused on the Health Hazard
Appraisal (HHA), which is also designed as an educational
self-help tool, focusing on the things people can do to help
themselves promote better health (Dunton and Elias, 1979;
Weiss, 1984). From over twenty years of data collection,
Jack Hall and Lewis Robbins, physicians from Methodist
Hospital of Indiana, developed the Health Hazard Appraisal
technique using the medical health model and the philosophy
of prospective medicine (Vogt, 1981; Smith-Shultz, 1984).

Most HHA instruments collect data on physical characteristics (height, weight, blood pressure), lifestyle factors (smoking, exercise), and the client's personal and family medical history. HHA is a system designed for the prevention of illness and the promotion of health through the stimulation of lifestyle change. It provides a framework in which to present health information, a task in which to involve the client, and personalized feedback which serves as a printed summary of the information collected (Milsum, 1980; Weiss, 1984). It is a technique in which individual health related behaviors and personal characteristics are compared to mortality statistics and epidemiologic data in order to estimate the risk of dying by some specified future time (usually ten years) along with the amount of risk which could be eliminated by making appropriate behavioral changes (Wagner et al, 1982).

Reasons that programs use HHA range from the view that HHA is a convenient and attractive instrument for the collection of data and to attract attention to one's program to the view of HHA as a powerful motivational medium for stimulating behavior change leading to reduction in illness and health care costs (Wagner et al, 1982). However, the effectiveness of HHA in promoting lifestyle change has been seriously questioned. Wagner et al (1982), reporting on three randomly controlled studies, notes that one study found no impact on attitudes and a second found no impact on health related behaviors. The findings of the third study, although it reports numerous behavior changes, should be viewed as only suggestive because of the subjects chosen (Canadian government workers). On the basis of this review, Wagner states that "the enthusiasm for HHA/HRA (health risk assessment) has been fueled by anecdotal reports of its effectiveness in increasing participation in health promotion programs and in motivating behavioral change"(p 351). Cioffi (1979), in a study designed to measure the effects of health status feedback on health beliefs reports that the manner of feedback did not influence health beliefs. She writes that intentions to perform the behavior are still the best predictors of the behavior, and that the Health Belief Model variables add little to prediction if intentions are measured as well.

Our instrument is not a Health Hazard Appraisal. We make no predictive statements about our respondents chances of injury, illness or death. In fact in the brochure which we send to respondents explaining cancer's warning signs and risk factors we clearly state, "Having a cancer warning sign or being at risk does not mean that you have or will get cancer. Nor does knowing these signs and risk factors mean you will not get cancer." Our instrument is a promotional device used to motivate individuals to become more (and better) informed of the risks for developing cancer and to increase awareness that there are things one can do to reduce the chances of developing cancer. A review of the literature indicates that most HHA's are administered in controlled environments (i.e. doctor's offices, health centers, school groups) and are targetted at one's "general" health (Lazlo, 1977; Fielding, 1982; Wagner et al, 1982). They are not, therefore, used as screening tools for existing disease, as is our instrument, and, indeed, pre-existing disease conditions typically invalidate the HHA risk assessment (Milsum, 1980). We compare our instrument with the health hazard/health risk appraisal instruments because of similarity of purpose, outreach and information in order to, as Dunton and Elias(1979) put it, "assist individuals in understanding their health risks and begin the reflective process of the way they live each day and learn that their behaviors may influence their overall health status"(p 31). The heart of our program is its educational component.

DEVELOPMENT OF "THE FIVE MINUTE CAN-DO HEALTH QUIZ

Through our contacts with a variety of community leaders we were able to convene focus groups in mid-1984. These groups contributed to the modification of the wording of the risk assessment instrument so that statements are expressed at an understandable reading level, are short and easy to answer, and are commonly understood by the target population, adults age twenty-five and older (Hunt et al, 1985).

The form covers eight sites: mouth and throat, breast (women), skin and lymph nodes, kidney and bladder, stomach and bowel, lung, male reproductive organs, and female reproductive organs. Questions are asked about current signs/symptoms of disease, personal medical history, family medical history, and personal risk factors (e.g. smoking or work exposure). Individuals can complete the form at home and mail it to the Center for analysis. A personalized letter is then sent to the respondents with specific recommendations along with a brochure explaining cancer risk factors and warning signs.

DESCRIPTION OF AREA/POPULATION

The Intervention area for our project consists of twenty-five adjacent census tracts. Of the over 100,000 residents, 99% are white and 47% are male. Approximately one-quarter of the residents are under the age of 18; 12% are between the ages of 18 and 24; 22% between 25 and 44; 24% between 45 and 64; and 16% are 65 years of age or older. The area is considered working class and has a median household income of $13,000 (Philadelphia City Planning Commission, 1982). A majority of the local residents have roots in the neighborhood which go back several generations. They have been described as traditional in their outlook, maintaining a skeptical view of educational and scientific programs and are said to be suspicious of the bureaucratic and technical appearance of health related services (Childers and Post, 1976; Workman, 1985).

METHODS

Two major methods for distribution of the CAN-DO Health Quiz were assessed; mail and person to person. Within these two methods we were interested in the influence of community support for participation in our program. For those mailed we compare participation by level of support for the program. For those distributed hand to hand we compare participation by the type of event, community-wide events or group meetings, and the level of support for the program.

In the spring of 1985 we distributed over 24,000 CAN-DO Quizzes, by mail, to five distinct geographical neighborhoods, each with their own formal organizational networks. Names and addresses for these mailings were purchased from a commercial mailing house. In two of these neighborhoods community links to our program were strong (in that they had good representation on the project's steering committee and had been blitzed by a promotional campaign in their local newspapers, banks, and shopping centers) whereas in the other three, links were either weak or absent. Results are presented in Table 1.

Two quizzes were sent to each household. The quiz return rate was calculated on the basis of 1980 census data which show that in the Intervention area, 48% of the households consist of a single adult (28% are single-person households and 20% are single headed households)

(Philadelphia City Planning Commission, 1982). Thus for each area the number of quizzes expected are 2444, 1278, 8003, 4358, and 2262, respectively.

Table 1

	Households Mailed To	Number of Quizzes Returned	Number of Households Returned	Quiz Return Rate	Household Return Rate
STRONG I	1608	350	235	14%	15%
WEAK II	841	126	94	10%	11%
STRONG III	5265	1291	896	16%	17%
WEAK IV	2867	544	391	12%	14%
WEAK V	1488	182	131	8%	9%

If we examine these figures in terms of community links to our program, it can be seen that we received a significantly better return rate in those areas where there was strong community support (see Table 2).

Table 2

	Households Mailed To	Number of Quizzes Returned	Number of Households Returned	Quiz Return Rate	Household Return Rate
Strong	6873	1641	1131	16%	16%
Weak	5196	852	616	11%	12%

p=0.0001

In the person to person distributions, quizzes were handed out: (1) at a "community-pride" fair in which local businesses and industries had displays and exhibits; (2) at a program-sponsored "Healthy Halloween" parade which served to draw attention to our program by bringing the family together in an enjoyable event with a healthy theme; and (3) at two local churches, following Mass. The priests in these churches were very supportive of our work and strongly encouraged their parishioners to complete the quiz. This last method was chosen on the recommendations of an external scientific review committee which firmly believed this method would prove extremely effective. These hand distributions also involved neighborhoods where ties to our program were strong and those where they were weak. These results are presented in Table 3.

Table 3

	Number Handed Out	Quizzes Returned	Households Returned	Quiz Return Rate
STRONG "Pride Day" Fair	579	90	78	16%
WEAK Church I	1499	136	121	9%
STRONG Halloween Parade	444	29	26	7%
WEAK Church II	1536	140	137	9%

If we again examine these figures in terms of community links to our program, it can be seen that we once again received a significantly better return rate in those areas where there was strong community support. These results are presented in Table 4.

As one can see from Table 3, a parade may not be an ideal situation for the distribution of health related materials. In our experience, the low response rate may be due to the nature of the parade (a children's Halloween parade) or to the mobile nature of parades in general which attract sightseers, not participators (although we did wait until we were assembled in a park, presenting prizes to the children, to distribute the quizzes). In any event, if we compare the return rates for "strong" versus "weak" ties, excluding the results from the parade, we get a return rate of 16% from the community with strong ties to our program and a 9% rate from those with weak ties.

Table 4

	Number Handed Out	Quizzes Returned	Households Returned	Quiz Return Rate
Strong	1023	119	104	12%
Weak	3035	276	258	9%

p=0.0107

Finally, if we compare the return rates for those mailed versus those distributed person to person, one can see that we received a significantly better return from those mailed.

Table 5

	Number Expected	Quizzes Returned	Households Returned	Quiz Return Rate
Mailed	18345	2493	1747	14%
Person to Person	4058	395	362	10%

p=0.0001

SUMMARY AND CONCLUSIONS

A person's decision to take part in a risk assessment program is based on two groups of factors: the attitudes and background unique to the individual, and his/her personal perception of its costs and benefits. Factors affecting the perceived costs and benefits include:

(1) fiscal responsibility;
(2) program availability, in terms of time and distance;

(3) fulfillment of higher priority needs (housing, nutrition) before risk assessment becomes acceptable;
(4) source credibility (Hsu and Milsum, 1978).

In examining the return rates we received, it is apparent that the percent of quizzes returned was not particularly high, regardless of the method of distribution or the level of community support. It must be remembered, however, that we are not distributing our quizzes in a controlled setting, as is done with most risk appraisal instruments, and that even in controlled settings return rates vary considerably. Johns (1976) reported that only 15% of a random sample of active patients completed and returned an HHA/HRA instrument which they had received in the mail. Studies reporting on the use of the Nottingham Health Profile yielded response rates ranging from 72% to 93%, but these were from highly motivated patient groups (Hunt et al, 1985). In addition, our target population consists of low income people. Weiss (1984) states that "for poor people, the urgency of immediate needs for physical and economic security relegates lifestyle behaviors and health habits to lower priority, and limitations in personal and societal resources constrain behavioral change opportunities." (p.281) In considering our response rates one must also keep in mind the numbers of quizzes returned and available for analysis. In less than nine months we have accumulated data on risk factors and warning signs for over 2800 adults. Other risk assessment programs cited in the literature process from a few dozen to 2000 cases, even after two years of operation (Dunton and Elias, 1979; Bartlett, 1983). If, as Laszlo (1977) says, the important factor is only that enough people respond so as to ensure a "ripple effect" or chain reaction of ever increasing size, then we are well on our way to reaching a significant portion of the community. He goes on to say that "the fact that only those who are already "half-sold" respond is perfectly satisfactory, since they will be the enthusiasts who will subsequently enthuse others." (p.28)

Designing and developing health promotion programs which target a specific disease and that draw on the community as a support structure requires a careful assessment of the image of disease held by the target population. Ben-Sira's (1977) discussion of the structure and dynamics of the image of diseases shows that the image held by community residents can

foster or impede the effectiveness of programs designed to
alter or enhance health practices and behaviors. Cancer,
like heart disease, is very much affected by lifestyle
factors. Doll and Peto (1981) estimate that tobacco usage
and inadequate diets are related to 30% and 35% of all cancer
deaths, respectively. If the image of cancer differs from
that of cardiovascular disease, the degree of readiness to
accept disease-specific health promotion programs may also
vary and may require alternative programming approaches. The
works of Mackie (1973) and Sloan and Gruman (1983) support
the notion that people do hold differing perceptions of the
two diseases, with those of heart disease being more
positive. A survey conducted in the target and a control
community to assess pre-intervention levels of cancer and
heart-disease related knowledge, attitudes and practices
confirm that the residents in each area do indeed have a more
positive image of heart disease (Amsel, Balshem and
Goldberg-Alberts, 1986).

Currently we are analyzing a follow-up to the CAN-DO
Quiz. We have interviewed a random sample of those who
responded to our quiz and of those who did not respond. We
are interested in perceptions about the instrument,
effectiveness of our risk appraisal letter in prompting
appropriate health related behaviors, and ways to improve
data collection procedures. Initial results are promising.
Sixty percent of those who received advice to see a physician
did so. Of these, 98% did so because of our advice.
Analysis of data from non-respondents indicates that a
majority did not recall receiving the quiz. However, of the
over 200 non-respondents we interviewed, 67% completed the
CAN-DO Quiz as part of the follow-up interview. Examination
of these indicate that non-respondents report fewer symptoms
than those who responded initially.

We are also intensifying our educational campaign aimed
at altering the image community residents hold regarding
cancer and attacking widely held misconceptions. In so doing
we hope to alter beliefs about cancer, increase awareness
that there are things that can be done to reduce the risk of
developing cancer, and thus increase the effectiveness of our
program.

REFERENCES

Amsel Z, Balshem AM, Goldberg-Alberts R (1986). The image of disease: Implications for health education programming for cancer and heart disease. Unpublished manuscript.

Bartlett EE, et al (1983). Health hazard appraisal in a family practice center: An exploratory study. J Comm Hlth 9(2):135-144.

Ben-Sira Z (1977). The structure and dynamics of the image of diseases. J Chron Dis 30:831-842.

Childers T, Post J (1976). The blue collar adult's information needs, seeking behavior and use: Final report. Unpublished manuscript, Drexel University School of Library Science.

Cioffi JP (1979). The effect of health status feedback on health beliefs: An inquiry into the prebehavioral outcomes of a health hazard appraisal. Proceedings of the 15th Annual Meeting on Prospective Medicine and Health Hazard Appraisal. Bethesda: Health and Education Resources:41-47.

Dayal H, et al (1984). Ecologic correlates of cancer mortality patterns in an industrialized urban population. JNCI 73(3):565-574.

Doll R, Peto R (1981). The Causes of Cancer. Oxford University Press.

Dunton S, Elias W (1979). Well aware about health: A controlled clinical trial of health assessment and behavior modification. Proceedings of the 15th Annual Meeting on Prospective Medicine and Health Hazard Appraisal. Bethesda: Health and Education Resources:31-38.

Farquhar JW (1978). The community-based model of life-style intervention trials. Amer J Epidemiol 108:103-111.

Faust HS, Vilnius D (1980). The effects of three health hazard appraisals on health beliefs and a comparative evaluation of three health hazard appraisals. Proceedings of the 16th Annual Meeting of the Society of Prospective Medicine:136-141.

Fielding JE (1982). Appraising the health of health risk appraisal. AJPH 72(4):337-340.

Hsu DHS, Milsum JH (1978). Impementation of health hazard appraisal and its impediments. Can J Pub Hlth 69:227-232.

Hunt SM, et al (1985). Measuring health status: a new tool for clinicians and epidemiologists. J R Coll Gen Pract April.

Johns RE (1976). Health hazard appraisal-A useful tool in health education? Proceedings of the 12th Annual Meeting of the Society of Prospective Medicine. Bethesda: Health and Education Resources.

Laszlo CA (1977). An integrated health hazard appraisal program: Applications, development and research. Proceedings of the 13th Meeting of the Society of Prospective Medicine. Bethesda: Health and Education Resources:27-30.

Mackie M (1973). Lay perception of heart disease in an Alberta community. Can J Pub Hlth 64:445-454.

Milsum JH (1980). Lifestyle changes for the whole person: Stimulation through health hazard appraisal. In Davidson PO, Davidson SM (eds): "Behavioral Medicine," New York: Brunner/Mazel, pp 116-150.

Philadelphia City Planning Commission. Selected Population and Housing Characteristics, 1980. Technical Information Paper, May 1982.

Puska P, et al (1983). Change in risk factors for coronary heart disease during 10 years of a community intervention program. Br Med J 287:1040-1044.

Sloan RP, Gruman JC (1983). Beliefs about cancer, heart disease and their victims. Psychol Rep 52(2):415-424.

Smith-Shultz CM (1984). Lifestyle assessment: A tool for practice. Nurs Clin N Amer 19(2):271-281.

Vogt TM (1981). Risk assessment and health hazard appraisal. Ann Rev Pub Hlth 2:31-47.

Wagner EH, et al (1982). An assessment of health hazard/ health risk appraisal. AJPH 72(4):347-352.

Weiss SM (1984). Health hazard/health risk appraisals. In Matarazzo JD, et al (eds): " Behavioral Health," New York, John Wiley and Sons, Inc., pp 275-294.

Workman S, et al (1985). Identifying and addressing health beliefs in the planning of a cancer control community intervention program. Unpublished paper. Presented at the Annual Health Conference of the Pennsylvania Public Health Association, State College, PA: October 10, 1985.

Advances in Cancer Control: The War on Cancer—
15 Years of Progress, pages 173–181
© 1987 Alan R. Liss, Inc.

MARKETING CANCER INFORMATION TO UNDER-UTILIZING COMMUNITIES:
AN INTERVENTION AND CONTROL STUDY OF A NEWSPAPER FEATURE

Carey Azzara, M.A., Kate Duffy, M.S., Lorenz
Finison, Ph.D., Susan Oehme, B.S., Elizabeth
Mallon, B.S., W. Bradford Patterson, M.D.

Dana-Farber Cancer Institute, 44 Binney Street
Boston, MA   02115

INTRODUCTION

The Cancer Communications System Office that serves
Massachusetts is part of a nationwide system of 16 offices
funded by the National Cancer Institute. Each office oper-
ates a free telephone service, the Cancer Information Service
(CIS), to provide accurate, up-to-date information on cancer
to patients, their families, health professionals and the
general public. In addition, every office is responsible
for developing cancer communication programs to meet identified needs in each service area.

The Massachusetts office is located at the Dana-
Farber Cancer Institute in Boston. This office produces
a Cancer Information Column (CIC) which appears weekly in
the Boston Sunday Globe. The content is based on questions
asked by Globe readers, common inquiries to the CIS, and
other current topics in cancer treatment and research. The
column appears in question and answer format and directs all
inquiries to the toll-free Cancer Information Service
number, 1-800-4-CANCER.

A previous analysis of the CIS call rates by city and
town showed that significant variation existed (Azzara,
et al, 1983). With few exceptions, the populations with
the lowest call rates were from older industrial cities
outside of the Boston mass media market. Cities with the
highest call rates were served by the Boston Globe. These
findings stimulated further investigation of the Cancer
Information Column's influence on call rates. Two studies

have been implemented and are described below. The first was a correlational study (Finison et al, 1983) and the second a field study with a quasi experimental design.

CIS OPERATIONS

Every call received by the CIS is entered on a call record form. Recorded information concerning each caller includes, but is not limited to: (1) zip code, (2) sex, (3) type of caller, e.g., consumer or health professional, (4) whether the caller has ever used the service before, and (5) how the caller first found out about the CIS. Consumers are defined as patients, persons with symptoms of cancer, significant others of patients or symptomatic persons, and the general public. These CIS consumers account for 57 percent of the first time callers and are clearly the largest audience and are of primary concern to the Cancer Communications System (CCS) office. The studies are confined to consumers who are first time callers to avoid problems of interpretation created by including previous users, health professionals, students, and all others.

STUDY I

Methods

Our data consists of all first time consumer calls from Massachusetts for the period July 1, 1982 to March 31, 1983. The call volumes for each city and town have been compared with 1980 U.S. Census data to generate call rates for each of the 351 communities in Massachusetts. In generating call rates, we used the numbers of households rather than individuals. This strategy resulted from the common observation that calls often come to the CIS from one household member (usually female) "representing" the information needs of the household. None of the conclusions of the present analysis would be substantively altered, however, by the alternative use of individuals in the denominators of our rates (the correlation between the two alternative measures is .98).

In addition to call rate data, we have obtained Census data on other characteristics of the cities and towns (e. g., percent of population 18 years of age and over), median income, percent with college education, percent Spanish origin) and data on the Boston Globe's circulation on March 9, 1982 (Audit Bureau of Circulations, 1982). These latter data have been combined with the Census household data to produce circulation rates for each city and town. We present these data below to develop a model for understanding the patterns of variation in call rates among Massachusetts communities.

Results

The first time consumer call rate for Massachusetts as a whole is slightly under 100 calls per 100,000 households for the first six month period reviewed. There is significant variation in this rate. Some very small communities show either very low rates (60 small communities, with under 1,000 households, had zero calls) or very high rates (16 other small communities had rates greater than 200 per hundred thousand). These variations may simply reflect sampling error, as demonstrated by the fact that aggregating the 30 smallest communities where individual rates show the greatest fluctuation gives an overall rate not significantly different from the state-wide average.

Of greater interest is the fact that there are several much larger communities which also produced very few calls. These low rates cannot be attributed to "sampling error" and suggest that large pockets of uninformed consumers may exist in Massachusetts. In order to report the results from these communities, the remainder of our analysis involves a subset of 108 Massachusetts cities and towns with more than 5,000 households. For this subset, the call rate varied between 19 and 256 per 100,000 households. Variation in call rate showed definite geographical patterning, association with Globe circulation, and association with various socio-demographic characteristics of the 108 communities.

With few exceptions, the populations with the lower rates were from older industrial cities. Cities with the highest call rates were served by the Boston Globe. The correlation matrix in Table 1 displays the relationships between each of these variables. It is clear from this Table that all four variables explain a reasonably high degree of the variance in call rates.

TABLE 1. Correlation Matrix of City Call rates with City
Demographic Data and Boston Globe circulation rates.

	CALL RATES	GLOBE RATES	INCOME	EDUCATION
GLOBE RATES	.71			
INCOME	.54	.64		
EDUCATION	.55	.65	.69	
HISPANIC	-.17	-.24	-.45	-.30

CALL RATES: CITY AND TOWN CALL RATES
GLOBE RATES: BOSTON GLOBE CITY CIRCULATION RATES
INCOME: MEDIAN HOUSEHOLD INCOME
EDUCATION: PERCENT WITH SOME COLLEGE EDUCATION
HISPANIC: PERCENT HISPANIC ORIGIN

Call rate is most highly associated with Globe circulation rates (r=+.71). The inverse association between percent Spanish origin and call rate is low and barely significant.. The association between median income and call rate
and percent college educated and call rate are substantial,
though lower than that between Globe circulation and call
rate. An association between "18 and over" and call rate
was also calculated, but was negligible (r=+.04).

Due to the high degree of colinearity among Globe
circulation, percent college educated, and median income,
the data were entered into a path analysis (Nie, et al,
1975) to estimate the strength of causal associations.

Path analysis requires the a priori development of a
"weak causal model." This model consists in the linking
of each item with each other item in the form x----> y.
The arrow is interpreted to mean: x may or may not affect
y but y cannot affect x. Each x and y in the model are then
linked by path coefficients showing the degree of direct
or causal connection. The path coefficients are the
standardized regression weights from the multiple regression
equations for each variable with every other variable having
weak causal linkage. The causal model and relevant path

coefficients are illustrated in Figure 1. The decomposition of covariation into causal and non-causal portions
is presented in Table 2.

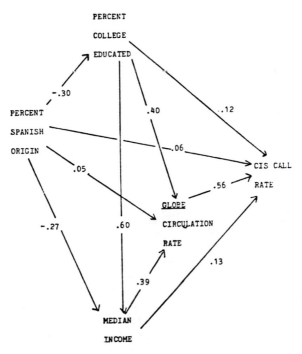

Figure 1. Path Analysis of Cancer Information Service Call
Rates for Massachusetts Cities and Towns with over 5000
Households

Table 2. Decomposition Table For CIS Call Data

Bivariate Relationship	Total Covariance	Causal			Noncausal
		Direct	Indirect	Total	
Spanish % with CIS Call Rate	-.17	.06	-.24	-.18	None
College % with CIS Rate	+.55	.12	.43	.55	None
Median Household Income with CIS call rate	+.54	.13	.22	.35	.19
Globe rate with CIS call rate	+.71	.56	None	.56	.15

STUDY II

Methods

To further test the hypothesis that the Cancer Information Column increases public awareness about cancer, it
was marketed to newspapers in areas with low call rates and
low Boston Globe circulation rates. We selected cities into
the study with: call rates less than 4 per 100,000 households and a population greater than 29,000. Cities served
by the same newspaper formed clusters and these news media
markets were used as the unit of intervention. Ten media
markets that met the above criteria were identified. They
were divided into matched intervention and control groups,
matched for similar call rates, city sizes and newspaper
circulation rates. To avoid potential contamination from
the intervention, control sites were selected for geographic isolation from newspapers serving the intervention
media markets. In September 1983 four editors agreed to
participate by publishing the Cancer Information Column on a
regular basis. One newspaper that refused was added to the
control group and its matched site was accrued into the
study, as an intervention site.

A publication history for all five newspapers was maintained that included the date of publication and the cancer topic. Call volumes for intervention, control, and all other Massachusetts cities and towns were collected from January 1983 through September 1985. The 9 month pre-intervention period from January through September 1983 was compared with the two 9 month post-intervention periods January to September 1984 and 1985.

Results

Call volumes have been steadily increasing over time at the Massachusetts CIS. During the pre and post period of this study calls to the CIS increased by 37.6 percent among the type of caller included in this analysis. The percent change in call volumes for intervention and control sites and all other communities are shown in Table 3.

Table 3. Percent Change in Call Volumes for Intervention and Control Groups and all other Massachusetts communities.

	PERCENT CHANGE			
	1983-84	95% CI	1983-85	95% CI
Intervention	42.4%	(37.2-47.7)	36.3%	(31.2-41.4)
Control	27.1%	(22.8-31.3)	15.9%	(12.4-19.4)
Other Communities	37.2%	(35.8-38.6)	40.9%	(39.4-42.4)

The percent increase in call volume for the intervention group is significantly higher than the increase for the control group. This held true for both 1984 and 1985. In fact the increase in the intervention group was similar to that among all other Massachusetts communities, while the control group lagged behind in both 1984 and 1985.

Data on how callers had first found out about the CIS was also examined. Since callers often have difficulty remembering where they first heard about the CIS these numbers are small. The results, however, indicate a clear trend.

Table 4. Comparison of Selected Ways Callers First Found
out About the Cancer Information Service

	CIC SPECIFIC			NEWSPAPER GENERAL		
	1983*	1984	1985	1983	1984	1985
Intervention	1	26	33	7	19	18
Control	3	4	1	25	27	25

* Globe CIC may have been read in the pre-intervention year.

The control group population appears to be reading about
the CIS in newspaper articles other than the Cancer Information Column, as much, if not more than those in the intervention group. Furthermore, its clear that the CIC had an
impact on the intervention population, while it remained
virtually unknown in the control population.

Discussion

The results of these studies argue for a significant
relationship between the publication of the Cancer Information Column and variation in CIS call volumes. The first
study indicates that there is significant variation in CIS
call rates associated with Boston Globe circulation rate,
median income, college educated and percent Spanish origin,
but not with percent age 18 and over. Arguments for a causal relationship between the Cancer Information Column and
CIS call volume rest on:
1. The partial correlation between call rate and Globe
circulation rate (causal r=.56);
2. The path analysis;
3. The significant change in the proportion of call volumes
demonstrated in the field experiment; and,
4. The evidence that callers in the intervention media markets did find out about the CIS directly from the CIC.
The fact that we could only link a small percent of calls
to the column directly suggests that it produces awareness that

is translated into action only when a household member is confronted with a need for cancer information. Awareness of the CIS may be passed on from one family member to another, or from friend to friend, therefore, the actual caller reports that they found out about the CIS from a source other than the column.

The results of the field study, although significant, were less dramatic than expected. This can be accounted for primarily by reviewing the publication history of the newspapers. The total number of published columns during the two 9 month post-intervention periods was N=81, which is less than one column per month per newspaper. There were, in fact, several months when one or more of the editors chose not to publish the column. We think the interuption in the publication schedule detracted from the impact of this intervention. Given the hypothesis that the CIC's effort depends on increasing and sustaining community's awareness of the CIS, consistent publication is essential. Future efforts to use this publicity tool should include more promotion of the column with editor's and their staff to ensure regular publication.

The implications of the results presented above are that such interventions will be necessary to adequately serve the large portion of the population which resides outside of major media markets. The application of our method of analysis to other health information services may provide valuable planning data on strategies for targeting promotional and educational efforts to communities in need.

REFERENCES

Azzara, C., et al. June 1983. The Cancer Information Service: Alternative methods for analyzing utilization. Association of American Cancer Institutes Conference.
Audit Bureau of Circulations, October 1982. ABC Audit Report, Boston Globe.
Finison, L., et al. October 1983. Marketing Cancer Information to under-utilizing communities. Unpublished.
Nie, N.H., et al. (1975). Statistical package for the social sciences. Second Edition, New York: McGraw-Hill.

Advances in Cancer Control: The War on Cancer—
15 Years of Progress, pages 183–187
© 1987 Alan R. Liss, Inc.

QUALITY ASSURANCE IN HOSPICE CARE

Barbara A. McCann
Director, Accreditation Program for Hospice Care
Joint Commission on Accreditation of Hospitals
Chicago, Illinois 60611

Robert E. Enck, M.D.
Director, Riverside Regional Cancer Institute
Riverside Methodist Hospital
Columbus, Ohio 43214

Quality assurance is a critical element of any health
care delivery system including the relatively new field of
hospice care. Both the Joint Commission on Accreditation of
Hospitals (JCAH) and the Medicare Hospice Benefit require
quality assurance programs as follows:

> JCAH: There is an ongoing quality assurance
> program designed to objectively and
> systematically monitor and evaluate
> the quality and appropriateness of
> patient/family care, pursue oppor-
> tunities to improve patient/family
> care and resolve identified problems.

> Medicare: A hospice must conduct an ongoing,
> comprehensive, integrated, self-assess-
> ment of the quality and appropriate-
> ness of care provided including in-
> patient care, home care and care pro-
> vided under arrangements.

As these requirements suggest, the quality assurance
program is self-directed with each individual hospice tail-
oring its own specific quality assurance program to meet
broad based principles. Quality assurance is a patient oriented program and strives to maintain the provision of high
quality care for each patient/family in hospice. It should
be viewed as educational and positive rather than as puni-
tive and negative which, unfortunately, occurs often. The
Joint Commission is introducing quality assurance to the
hospice field for several reasons important to the manage-

ment and improvement of hospice care.

Quality assurance is a process that provides useful information concerning the utilization and appropriateness of service, as well as the quality of care given. The information gathered is such that it becomes useful to program directors in assuring

1. the clinical competence of staff;
2. the appropriate and cost effective use of resources;
3. compliance with federal and state regulations;
4. risk management;
5. provision of appropriate information to the governing body, if the program is providing good care and meeting designated goals.

Where to begin quality assurance depends on the answer to two simple questions:

1. What are high volume patients and services?
2. What are high risk patients and services?

When these questions have been answered, the hospice staff is able to determine what aspects of care to monitor. Quality assurance involves developing a system for monitoring aspects of care which will continuously identify problems and opportunities for improving care. It is also important to designate who has the authority to implement the quality assurance plan and who will assume the responsibility for these activities. A committee may be used to implement this quality assurance plan but the hospice staff should use caution when appointing interdisciplinary team members to the quality assurance committee because it may only increase their time demands and frustrations.

When the broad areas of care to monitor have been identified, then indicators must be developed. These statements indicate quality or appropriate care in hospice. For example, nursing is a key high volume and high risk service. Therefore, an indicator of good hospice nursing care may be:

An appropriate pain and symptom assessment of all patients is performed by an RN within 24 hours of admission.

Following the establishment of an indicator, the interdisciplinary team or committee then develop criteria. Criteria are measurable statements of acceptable practice in the hospice program. Hospice nurses set the peer criteria for each other; program standards are based on acceptable clinical practice. The following are some examples of criteria:

1. There is a pain and symptom assessment by an RN in 100 percent of the patients' charts within 24 hours of admission. Exception - patients admitted between 6 p.m. on Fridays and 8 a.m. on Mondays.

2. The assessment includes: a total physical systems review; notation of the current location, frequency and intensity of pain; current medications; effectiveness of medications; patient/family understanding of regimen and compliance.

3. All patients/families are given a pain questionnaire two weeks after admission. Sixty-five percent of the patients should respond that their pain is adequately managed and they are comfortable.

Depending on staff comfort with quality assurance and the care process, only one of the criteria or all three may be used. For example, in one hospice documentation may be a problem, and the staff may spend six months just assuring that the completed assessment form is in the record. Another hospice, one that is secure with their documentation and assessment process, may be ready to address the question of the effectiveness of their pain management program by dealing directly with patient outcomes by means of a questionnaire.

Another area may involve the attending physician and pain control. A physician advisory committee is formed to establish an indicator and criteria. An indicator of pain control by the attending physician may be:

Acceptable pain control is achieved during the course of an inpatient admission.

The following are some examples of criteria:

1. Pain control is assessed on admission as noted in the history and physical examination as well as on a daily basis.

2. Changes in drugs employed, dosages, intervals or routes of administration, that is, from PO to SQ/IM or decreasing frequency of administration.

3. Readmission for pain control within
   48-72 hours excluding readmissions
   because of patient/family noncompliance.
4. Ongoing documented communication
   between the attending physician and the
   interdisciplinary team.

As in the previous example, only a few or all of these criteria may be utilized.

At least quarterly review of the results of the monitoring activities are recommended. While retrospective data is helpful in the beginning to appreciate trends in care, concurrent review allows changes in the patient care process to help patients/families currently in the program. The sources of data for the monitoring system should not be limited solely to chart review which provides information on only one dimension of the staff's care. Data retrieval should include a process where it is known, for example, whether or not a chart met the criteria, and also if each nurse responsible for the documentation, met the criteria over several charts.

Many programs have reduced the staff burden of quality assurance by training volunteers to review charts against criteria. In this way, the staff and management time is best used in responding to the results of the review and to implement action.

At any point when a discrepancy exists between what is expected and actual performance, the quality assurance committee must plan action to address the problem. For example, the initial chart review for nursing and the follow-up visits indicate that less than 60 percent of the patients admitted have an assessment which meets the criteria established. The quality assurance committee initiates the following action with appropriate persons who have authority in the program:

1. Patient care coordinator is notified of
   results and meets with home care nurses
   to reaffirm that criteria are valid.
2. Patient care coordinator and team nurses
   meet to re-format assessment sheet to
   include all criteria; quality assurance
   committee approves form.
3. Quality assurance committee advises
   patient care coordinator that present

        policy and procedure are inadequate
and does not verify process created;
patient care coordinator and team meet
and re-draft policy and procedure.
4. Medical director conducts inservice on
pain and symptom assessment.

All of the above actions are reports in second quarters
minutes of the quality assurance committee meetings.

Additional quality assurance functions include on-going monitoring with the criteria developed for each indicator to determine if the problems have been corrected or improved. The results of these quality assurance activities such as nursing and attending physician pain control may form the bases for programs such as inservice nursing education or medical staff presentations on pain control.

Quality assurance helps prevent costly repetition of inefficient assessment processes, sets clear expectations, and helps set realistic goals in care planning. But perhaps, most important, it encourages the establishment of national practice standards to assure quality differences in hospice care to the dying.

TRENDS IN COMMUNITY CANCER PROGRAMS

Advances in Cancer Control: The War on Cancer—
15 Years of Progress, pages 191–203
© 1987 Alan R. Liss, Inc.

CURRENT AND FUTURE CANCER CONTROL ACTIVITIES IN CANCER PROGRAMS IN THE UNITED STATES*

Zili Amsel, Sc.D.
Paul F. Engstrom, M.D.
Barbara Rimer, Dr.P.H.
Martha K. Keintz, Sc.M.
Doris Gillespie

Fox Chase Cancer Center
Philadelphia, PA 19111

BACKGROUND

The National Cancer Institute (NCI) has set a clear goal of reducing cancer deaths by 50% in the United States by the year 2000. The program being launched is intended to increase funding for smoking cessation and dietary change programs to reduce smoking by 1990 and to modify diets to include more fiber and less fats by 2000, and, to offer more extensive public education and related research programs to provide information about cancer detection and treatment. Over the past fifteen years, the federal government has established vehicles to fund a variety of programs designed to address the prevention and treatment of cancer. These programs are distributed across the country and parallel areas exhibiting high cancer mortality rates (as can be seen in Figures 1 and 2). These programs serve as resources to help NCI meet its year 2000 goals. To what extent do the activities performed by these programs address the NCI goals?

In a first-level inquiry into this question, the Cancer Control staff of the Fox Chase Cancer Center, in cooperation with the American Association of Cancer Institutes (AACI) and the Association of Community Cancer Centers (ACCC), sent surveys to 314 cancer programs in the United States (cancer institutes are differentiated from community cancer centers

* Supported by NCI-PHS Grant #CA34856.

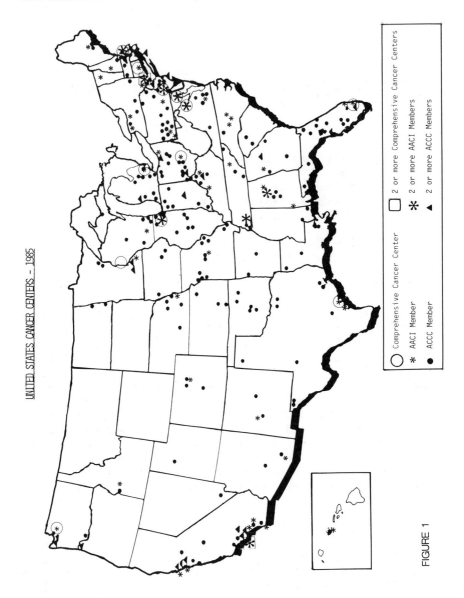

UNITED STATES CANCER CENTERS – 1985

Comprehensive Cancer Center ○   2 or more Comprehensive Cancer Centers □

AACI Member *   2 or more AACI Members *

ACCC Member ●   2 or more ACCC Members ▲

FIGURE 1

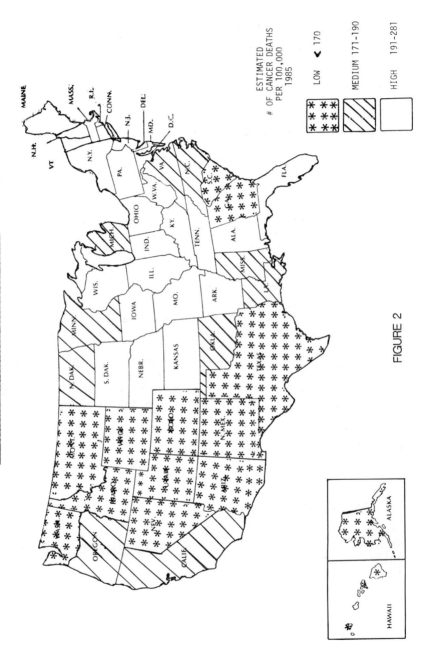

ESTIMATED # OF CANCER DEATHS PER 100,000 - 1985

ESTIMATED
OF CANCER DEATHS
PER 100,000
1985

LOW   ∨ 170

MEDIUM 171-190

HIGH   191-281

FIGURE 2

in that they are primarily research centers). A listing of these programs was compiled from the mailing lists of these two associations. Duplicate members were excluded from the ACCC list and assigned to AACI.

MATERIALS AND METHODS

The survey form sent out to the cancer programs consisted of three pages. Included in the survey form were questions about staffing of cancer control activities, amount and sources of funding for cancer control activities, current cancer control service and research activities, and for each activity, the targetted group, funding source, and expected level of funding by source over the next five years. Cancer control activities (Table 1) include the areas of prevention, detection and screening, diagnosis and treatment, rehabilitation and continuation of care and epidemiological research.

TABLE 1

Cancer Control Activities

Prevention

Smoking Cessation and
   Prevention
Chemoprevention
Dietary Modification
Exposure to Sunlight
Occupational Exposure
Professional Education

Detection and Screening

Cervix
Breast
Colon-Rectum
Skin
Professional Education

Diagnosis and Treatment

Dissemination of Protocols
Patient Education
Patterns of Care
Professional Education

Rehabilitation and
   Continuing Care

Psychosocial Activities
Professional Education

Epidemiological Research

After three mailings and a telephone follow-up, we received responses from 86% (or 270) of the programs; 91% from the cancer institutes and 85% from the community cancer centers. Of these 270 responding programs, 69% (or 186) stated they had some type of cancer control activity; the same percentage (69%) from both groups. (Table 2)

TABLE 2

Cancer Centers	Number Sent	Percent Returned
AACI	65	91
ACCC	249	85
Both	314	86

An overview of the types of cancer activities performed by the AACI and ACCC programs indicates that 42% offer smoking cessation services, 40% offer patient education services, 38% have psychosocial services, about one-third offer detection and screening for breast and colo-rectal cancer, and 30% disseminate treatment protocols. (Table 3)

Of the 130 programs for which information is most complete, we found that 17% (or 22) considered their cancer control activities to be mostly research-related, 27% (or 35) considered their activities to be primarily service, and the remaining 56% (or 73) reported both service and research activities. (Table 4)

The relationship of these activities and the characteristics that differentiate these three types of programs are the topics of this paper. Factors that are examined include geographic location, funding sources, staffing patterns, types of activities performed and types of populations being targetted for these activities.

RESULTS

Using the Standard Federal Regions as a guide, the programs were classified into 10 areas. These were collapsed into six areas: northeast, southeast, midwest, central, southwest and northwest. Table 5 shows the distribution of the 130 programs with the most complete information.

TABLE 3

Types of Cancer Control Service and Research
Activities Provided by Cancer Programs
in the United States - 1985 (Percentages)

	Service Activities	Research Activities
Total Number of Programs Activities	(186)	(186)
Prevention		
Smoking Prevention & Cessation	42	17
Chemoprevention	6	8
Diet Modification	19	10
Occupational Exposure	9	8
Professional Education	34	--
Detection and Screening		
Cervix	23	9
Breast	33	17
Colon-Rectum	32	12
Skin	14	5
Professional Education	28	--
Diagnosis and Treatment		
Dissemination of Protocols	30	34
Patient Education	40	18
Patterns of Care	19	19
Professional Education	37	--
Rehabilitation and Continuing Care		
Psychosocial Activities	38	19
Professional Education	27	--
Epidemiological Research	--	19

TABLE 4

Type of Cancer Control Program

	Number	Percent
Research only	22	17
Service only	35	41
Research and Service	73	56
All	130	100

TABLE 5

Type of Cancer Control Program by
Geographic Location (Percentage by Type of
Activities/Percentage by Geographic Location)

Type of Cancer Control Program

Geographic Location	Research Only	Service Only	Research and Service	All
Northeast	18/18	14/23	18/59	17
Southeast	36/20	34/30	27/50	31
Midwest	4/4	20/29	22/67	18
Central	14/16	11/21	16/63	15
Southwest	18/22	17/33	11/44	14
Northwest	9/29	3/14	5/57	5

Almost one-third of these programs are located in the southeastern United States while only 5% are located in the northwest. The remaining programs are distributed almost equally among the other areas. Examination of the three types of cancer control programs (those with research activities only, with service activities only and with both activities) indicates that there are fewer 'research only' programs in the midwest but more combined service and research programs. The presence of more combined programs also is seen for programs located in the central areas of the country.

Sources of funding include the federal government, state and local governments and other, primarily institutional or private foundations. It can be seen in Table 6 that most of the programs do not depend on one source of funding for their cancer control activities.

Over half have access to all three sources for their funds. Those programs performing both research and service activities are more likely to have funding from federal, state/local governments as well as institutional and private foundations. Programs that offer only service activities tend to have only one source of funding. In Table 7 the three types of cancer programs are examined by actual source of funding.

TABLE 6

Type of Cancer Control Program by Number
of Funding Sources Mentioned (Percentages)

Type of Cancer Control Program

	Research Only	Service Only	Research and Service	All
One mention	29	46	19	28
Two mentions	23	6	19	16
Three mentions	48	49	62	56
Average number mentioned	1.3	2.0	2.4	2.3

TABLE 7

Type of Cancer Control Programs
By Funding Source(s) (Percentages)

Type of Cancer Control Program

Funding Sources	Research Only	Service Only	Research and Service	All
Federal only	19	6	1	5
Federal & State	5	3	3	3
Federal & other	14	0	8	7
Federal, State, & other	48	49	62	56
State only	0	0	11	6
State & other	5	3	1	2
Other only	10	40	14	20

It can be seen that many more of the 'service only'
programs have their support from the "other only" category,
whereas the 'research only' programs are more likely to have
support from federal grants.

Another area of interest is staffing patterns. We asked
about the number of full-time equivalent doctoral and masters
level staff that are involved in the cancer control
activities. (Table 8) Thirty-five percent of the programs

have at least one full-time equivalent doctoral level staff person and 40%, at least one full-time masters level staff person. Many more of the programs with research activities, with or without service activities, have either one or more doctoral or masters level professionals than do the programs with cancer control services only.

TABLE 8

Type of Cancer Control Program
By Staffing Patterns (Percentages)

Staffing Patterns (full-time equivalents)	Type of Cancer Control Program			
	Research Only	Service Only	Research and Service	All
Doctoral level	41	17	41	35
Masters level	50	23	52	44

Examination of the three types of cancer programs by types of activities shows some variation across programs. There is a great deal of information contained in these tables, therefore this discussion will focus only on those activities that relate directly to the Year 2000 goals: smoking cessation/prevention, dietary modification and the screening and detection of cancers of the breast, cervix and colon/rectum.

It can be seen in Table 9 that most of the programs, within each type, perform activities related to smoking cessation and prevention. More of the 'service only' programs offer these activities than either of the other program types.

Within the programs that offer both service and research activities, 20% have combined research and service related to smoking cessation while 47% have only service activities.

Almost 40% of all programs offer 'dietary modification' activities. Examination of the combined service and research program indicate that 64% of the dietary modification activities are primarily research.

TABLE 9

Type of Cancer Related Program By
Type of Year 2000-Related Activity (Percentages)

Activity	Research Only	Service Only	Research and Service
Prevention			
Smoking prevention and cessation	59	86	72
Dietary modification	36	40	38
Screening and Detection			
Cervix	27	48	40
Breast	54	57	63
Colon-Rectum	45	60	57

Differences are noted in the screening and detection activities across program categories. More of the programs that have a service component tend to offer cervical and colo/rectal screening whereas these activities for breast cancer tend to be evenly distributed across categories. If we focus on the 'combined research and service' programs, we find most of the screening programs are considered to be research operations.

Lastly, Tables 10 and 11 present the cancer control activities by target population. The variable for 'population' is defined as a geographic or catchment area: state/region, other geographic subarea, demographic subarea, several institutions and one institution. It can be seen that most of the Year 2000 Goal-related activities are directed to large areas and, presumably, large population groups.

SUMMARY AND CONCLUSIONS

In summary, a preliminary survey was conducted among cancer programs to determine the status of cancer control activities in the United States and to assess these in light of the Year 2000 goals of the NCI. The initial examination of survey findings of 314 cancer programs (members of AACI and ACCC), showed that 69% of the 270 responding programs had at least one cancer control activity. Prominant among the

activities being offered are smoking prevention/cessation,
patient education, psychosocial services, screening and detection for breast and colo-rectal cancer and dissemination
of treatment protocols. Further examination of the survey
forms for 130 programs, for which complete information was
available, indicated that approximately 17% considered their
activities to be mostly research, 27% considered them to be
primarily service, and 56% reported both service and research

TABLE 10

Type of Cancer Control Program by
Target Population for Year 2000-Related Activities -
Prevention (Percentages)

Activity/Target Population	Type of Cancer Control Program		
	Research Only	Service Only	Research and Service
Smoking Prevention and Cessation			
State/Region	31	28	45
Other geographic sub area	15	31	25
Demographic sub group	15	10	6
Within several institutions	23	0	10
Within one institution	15	31	14
Dietary Modification			
State/Region	37	43	35
Other geographic sub area	12	21	23
Demographic sub group	12	7	11
Within several institutions	25	0	8
Within one institution	12	29	23

activities. Several factors were available for examination
to determine differences among these three types of programs:
geographic location, source of funding, staffing patterns and
type of activity. It was found that there was inequitable
distribution of programs across the country with fewer
overall programs located in the northwest and fewer 'research
only' programs in the midwest. In addition, it was found

that funding for these programs was diversified with most of the programs receiving funds from more than one source. Research activities tend to receive their support from federal sources whereas service activities, without research, receive support from "other" sources, either private foundations or home institutions. Research programs were also found to be more likely to have full-time equivalent doctoral and masters level staff.

TABLE 11

Type of Cancer Control Program by
Target Population for Year 2000-Related Activities –
Screening and Detection (Percentages)

| | Type of Cancer Control Program | | |
Activity/Target Population	Research Only	Service Only	Research and Service
Cervix			
State/Region	50	12	46
Other geographic sub area	17	59	25
Demographic sub group	0	6	11
Within several institutions	17	0	7
Within one institution	17	23	11
Breast			
State/Region	36	25	51
Other geographic sub area	27	50	23
Demographic sub group	18	5	5
Within several institutions	0	0	5
Within one institution	18	20	16
Colon/Rectum			
State/Region	60	30	55
Other geographic sub area	0	45	22
Demographic sub group	20	10	5
Within several institutions	10	0	5
Within one institution	10	15	12

Activities and their target populations were examined only for those activities that were directly related to the Year 2000 goals for NCI: smoking cessation/prevention,

dietary modification and the screening and detection of
cancers of the breast, cervix and colon/rectum. More of the
service programs provided these activities. Some differences
were noted across program types with most of the service
programs offering smoking cessation and cervical and
colo/rectal screening and more of the research programs
offering dietary modification and breast screening
activities. The majority of all the programs are targotting
large population groups.

Obviously, many of the smoking prevention/cessation and
dietary modification services available in the United States
are provided through auspices other than cancer programs and
may be funded to a greater extent from federal sources.
However, it appears that federal efforts to support research
rather than direct service activities have forced programs
with cancer control activities to seek other resources for
funding. Although there are positive features associated
with this phenomenon, it may have long term detrimental
effects:

1. Cancer programs will be competing for scarce
   funds particularly as research grants and
   contracts terminate, forcing programs to look
   for alternative funding.

2. Reduced service activities associated with
   research may suffer in quality and may be forced
   to limit the size of their target populations.

3. Service activities may be completely eliminated
   despite their level of effectiveness.

4. Poorer areas, and perhaps areas at most risk,
   may have fewer services available.

For these reasons, the cancer programs in conjunction
with federal, state and local governmental agencies should
develop a comprehensive plan for retaining existing programs
and adding new programs in areas of need. Guidelines
regarding creative alternative funding options should also be
compiled for cancer control program directors. With threats
of cut-backs, DRG's and limited third-party benefits, cancer
control services may not be available for those who need them
most and we may not be able to meet Year 2000 goals.

Advances in Cancer Control: The War on Cancer—
15 Years of Progress, pages 205-212
© 1987 Alan R. Liss, Inc.

EVALUATION OF THE IMPACT OF A CCOP PROGRAM IN A LOW
POPULATION DENSITY AREA OF MONTANA.

Neel Hammond, M.D., Ben Marchello, M.D.,
David Myers, M.D., Sandra Kampen, R.N.

Billings Interhospital Oncology Project
Grant # CA 325274-04

INTRODUCTION

The Billings Interhospital Oncology Project is
a Community Clinical Oncology Program (CCOP) which serves
a direct community of 90,000 people in Billings, Montana
plus a tertiary referral population of 400,000 in northern
Wyoming, eastern Montana, and portions of the Dakotas.
Our widely-spread area and extensive cancer control
experience prior to CCOP funding in 1983 make our program
an ideal one to evaluate for community impact. We set
about this by establishing a data base covering 432
patients entered on 519 studies over a 6 year period
from 1977 through 1983. We have compared this with
our CCOP experience, which is constituted by 222 patients
entered on 238 protocols through the first part of 1986.
We have additionally looked at 2 other data bases including ICD 9 codes for our two hospitals and our CCOP log
required by the National Cancer Institute. Our findings
clearly show the CCOP's ability to 1) select patients
whose data is more meaningful because of a decrease in
early death rate; 2) comply with a much more stringent
quality assurance from our major research base (the Southwest Oncology group); 3) succeed in increasing overall
accrual rates on a per month basis; and finally, 4) reach
outlying areas in our catchment through the use of clinics
established in communities of greater than 10,000 population. This report will demonstrate those impacts on
the data bases described.

METHODS: We used data bases including patients entered
on NCI-approved studies for both the pre and post-CCOP
era. We also maintain a CCOP log according to specifica-
tions outlined by the National Cancer Institute, and
finally, we looked at our respective hospitals' ICD
9 codes 140-240 for comparison purposes involving our
respective populations. In looking at those pre and
post-CCOP data bases, as well as the general patient
population data bases from both the hospital and the
CCOP log, we tried to establish differences in make-up
and outcome of those populations. The major questions
which were posed included: 1) Was the population any
different pre or post-CCOP? 2) Was the disease population
of patients entered on study significantly different
from either our hospital data or the CCOP log data base?
3) Were the research bases any different pre or post-CCOP?
4) What was the amount of data management change over
the 7 years of clinical cancer research? 5) What was
the change in type and number of accruals? (raw numbers,
locations, early death, etc.) 6) What did those changes,
if present, signified pre and post-CCOP?

RESULTS: A summary of our patient distribution is
shown in the first illustrated graph labeled Regional
Patient Distribution, which shows an increased percentage
of outlying patients who were actually entered on CCOP
as well as pre-CCOP studies. We felt this indicated
added availability to non-Billings and Wyoming patients
and felt this distribution to be a significant verification
of our research effort.

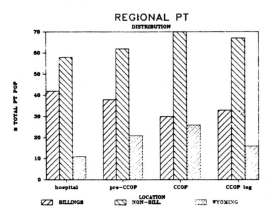

The accrual of patients on studies did increase post–CCOP from approximately 6 patients per month to a little over 8 patients per month, as illustrated in the second table.

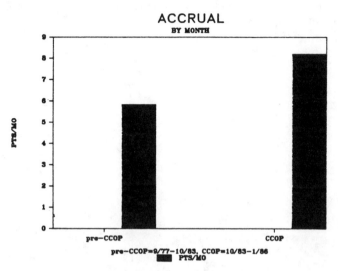

The influence of our outlier clinics was illustrated pre and post–CCOP by an increase of the percent of patients entered on studies from approximately 2½% of our total to over 9% of our total from the first community in which we established an outlying clinic (Sheridan, Wyoming).

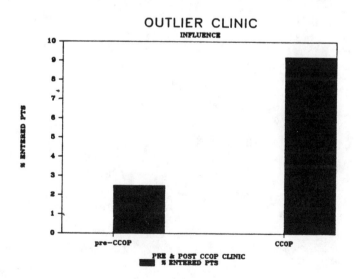

The National Cancer Institute, when funding of CCOP's began, expressed an interest in randomized questions among strictly defined patient populations rather than entry on pilot studies. We subsequently looked at the number of patients entered on our research bases and found that the relative percentage of patients entered on NSABP studies increased while those entered on University Cancer Center studies decreased.

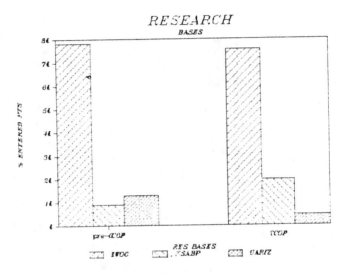

We additionally looked at disease distribution in which patients entered on studies among breast cancer, Hodgkin's disease, non-Hodgkin's lymphoma, acute leukemia, and test-ticular cancer were over-represented, as we had hoped, when compared to the hospital data base and CCOP log.

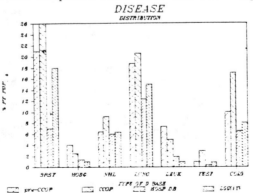

With the large amount of prior cancer control experience
we had to deal with increasing numbers of patients who were
long-term survivors and required ongoing data management,
dating back to our initiation of studies in 1977. We looked
at this in the following graph which shows the numbers of
patients we were following as of January the 1st of each
of the respective years. You will note that that number
has gone from 10 on January 1, 1979, to over 300 as of January 1, 1986.

PATIENTS
FOLLOWED

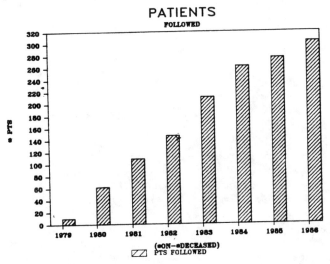

(●ON-●DECEASED)
▨ PTS FOLLOWED

Another method of looking at our entries on studies involved a more careful look at the CCOP log with respect to the
subspecialties represented in our community. The next graph
illustrates the extremely high percentage of entries on
study by both our surgical and medical oncologists who had
direct specialty research bases, as opposed to our radiation oncologists who had no direct specialty research base
affiliation and were subsequently not as directly involved
in patient entries. As you will note, of our patients
who had a protocol available, more than 70% were entered
on study by the medical oncologists and the surgical oncologist, whereas that figure drops to less than 10% with
our radiation oncologists.

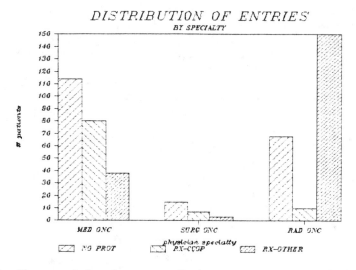

Finally, we felt that one of the major impacts of the
CCOP grant was an improved selection on study by the
research bases. We felt this was a significant question
in that the restrictions on our patient entries on phase
II studies changed dramatically with the onset of the
CCOP grant. We subsequently decided to look at two populations, patients who died in less than one month after
entry on study and patients dying in less than 3 months
from the date of entry on study. The next table shows
those figures pre and post-CCOP and a dramatic change in
those percentages is appreciated.

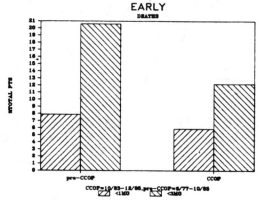

The types of tumors and the types of study entries would appear to reflect more closely whether patient selection really accounted for that. We looked at the characteristics of early death with respect to both primary tumor site and phase of study. As the next graphic illustrates, the majority of patients with early deaths were made up of far-advanced, poor-prognosis lung and colorectal cancer. Greater than 40 vs. less than 5 phase II entries experienced early deaths. Because of the fact that the same investigators were caring for these patients both pre and post-CCOP, we see this as direct evidence of selectivity with the onset of the CCOP grant.

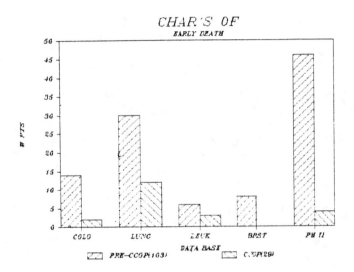

CHAR'S OF
EARLY DEATH

CONCLUSIONS: In summary, our CCOP has shown improved diffusion of state-of-the art cancer care in a low-population density area. We have shown that clinics in outlying areas does add to accrual, both in numbers and in regional distribution. We have additionally shown that control randomized studies and selection of phase II questions can be accomplished within the framework of a CCOP. Questions related to disease site, performance status, and type of study selection can be controlled within such a program. Finally, we have shown that a long-term data accrual process in the community can be achieved through a CCOP program with continuing quality data retrieval over 9 years of clinical cancer research experience. We feel the CCOP investment is an extremely worthwhile effort and hope that this data illustrates that.

Our goals for the future include: 1) maintenance of quality assurance within our research base framework, 2) expansion of our outlying clinic structure, 3) the addition of cancer control programs among both defined patient populations within the framework of our treatment protocols and well-subject recruitment and 4) establishment of an affiliation with regional centers in an attempt to answer larger questions in this low-population density area.

Advances in Cancer Control: The War on Cancer—
15 Years of Progress, pages 213–216
© 1987 Alan R. Liss, Inc.

GREEN MOUNTAIN ONCOLOGY GROUP - CCOP: AN EVOLVING REGIONAL
CANCER PROGRAM

H. James Wallace, Jr., M.D., John Valentine, M.D.
Mary Lou Giddings, R.N., O.C.N., Mark A. Donavan, M.D.
and Mildred A. Reardon, M.D.

Rutland Regional Medical Center, Rutland, Vermont 05701
(H.J.W. & M.L.G.) Central Vermont Hospital, Berlin, VT
(J.V.), Southwestern Vermont Medical Center, Bennington,
VT (M.A.D.) and Medical Center Hospital of Vermont,
Burlington, VT (M.A.R.)

The Green Mountain Oncology Group - CCOP (GMOG) was
formed in 1982 as a state-wide consortium of community oncologists who wished to work in close cooperation with The
University of Vermont/Vermont Regional Cancer Center (VRCC)
to enhance the accessibility of Vermonters to more sophisticated cancer treatments. There were four non-university
oncologists practicing in Vermont who were interested in
participating in clinical research trials and in responding
to the Community Clinical Oncology Program Request for Ap
plications. The four oncologist organized as a regional
cooperative group using the four largest hospitals in Vermont as the center of activities and influencing the care
of about 75% of cancer patients in the state. The Rutland
Regional Medical Center, a 300 bed community hospital in
Rutland was the primary institution with the Operations
Office and Data Management Center under the direction of
the Principal Investigator and Group Chairman. The other
participating institutions were the 175 bed Central Vermont Hospital in Berlin, the 180 bed Southwestern Vermont
Medical Center in Bennington and the 510 bed Medical Center Hospital of Vermont, the university hospital in Burlington (Fig.I). There are 12 other hospitals in Vermont, all
less than 100 beds.

The GMOG maintained a close relationship with Vermont
Regional Cancer Center as the primary research base and also
became a member of The Eastern Cooperative Oncology Group
and The National Surgical Adjuvant Breast and Bowel Project as additional primary research bases.

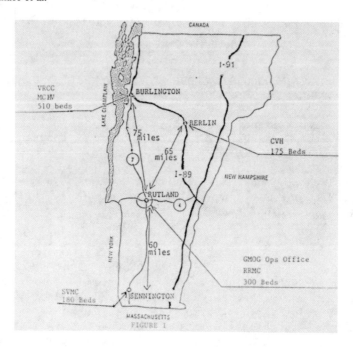

FIGURE 1

The University of Vermont previously had traditional out-reach programs such as tumor boards and cancer conferences at several hospitals and community oncologists occasionally participated in cooperative group clinical trials. There was, however, no formally organized program. The GMOG–CCOP greatly expanded the out-reach impact of the University by providing an organized support vehicle for the community oncologists so that they could more effectively participate in clinical cooperative trials.

The basic objective of the Community Clinical Oncology Program is being realized with significant contributions to NCI approved cooperative group protocols. Organizational problems slowed the first year activities but since then GMOG has met accrual goals with 72 credits in year two and 37 credits in the first six months of year three. These accrual goals have been reached without active lung cancer and first line breast cancer protocols available for the last year. To fill these gaps the Group is participating in selected protocols with Adria Laboratories for patients without higher priority NSABP or ECOG protocols.

The diffusion of the latest cancer treatment knowledge throughout the community is one of the key goals of the CCOP. However, the validity of the diffusion hypothesis has been difficult to assess. The GMOG was randomly assigned (without informed consent) to the Community Cancer Care Evaluation Patterns of Care Study which had the major objective of proving the hypothesis. The results of this study are pending. Diffusion, however, is clearly demonstrated and documented in more complete but focused diagnostic and staging sequences and a greater multidisciplinary participation in treatment planning for patients, whether they are entered on clinical trials or not. At Rutland Regional Medical Center each newly diagnosed patient is presented at the weekly tumor board for multidisciplinary discussion and considered for protocol eligibility.

The most significant objective changes which can be ascribed to the GMOG-CCOP are 1. The development of specialized oncology personnel and 2. The evolving regionalization of oncology resources. The requirements for complex protocol compliance and data management necessitated significant changes in clinical practice habits of physicians and required the training of specialized personnel not previously needed in the traditional community hospital oncology practice. Participation in the GMOG-CCOP protocols and The Patterns of Care Study has led to the development of a highly skilled Oncology Research Nurse/Administrator and a Data Manager who carry out the bulk of the day-to-day operation of the Group and assist the oncologists and their regular office staff in keeping good data flow on protocol patients. There is significant carry-over in data management for non-protocol patients which increases the quality of their care as well.

Regionalization of medical oncology personnel and resources for protocol participation has been accomplished through cooperative efforts establishing a good network for communications. This network has been the stimulus to begin important regionalization of other major resources; particularly a state-wide plan to provide radiation therapy of the highest quality. Presently the only radiation therapy facility in Vermont is at MCHV in Burlington and it is approaching current capacity. GMOG institutions in Rutland, Berlin, and Bennington are all more than one hour away from radiation therapy units in Burlington, Hanover, New Hampshire, Troy and Glens Falls, New York over highways which are rated by federal standards as poor to fair. An additional problem is that Vermont has no regulatory control over costs in these out of state treatment facilities.

Estimates of national utilization of radiation therapy indicate that 50% of cancer patients will benefit from radiation therapy sometime during the course of their disease. Rural communities such as Rutland are successfully referring only 30% of the patients for radiation therapy because they are denied easy access to these resources. The Rutland Regional Medical Center and The Medical Center Hospital of Vermont have joined together to bring high quality radiation therapy consultation and treatment closer to the patients who need it but find travel difficult or impossible. These two institutions have jointly sponsored a feasibility study which has resulted in the submission to the State Health Department of a Certificate of Need Application for a satellite radiation therapy program at RRMC as part of a Comprehensive Community Cancer Center. The proposed Community Cancer Center will bring together all of the cancer diagnostic and treatment modalities as well as the necessary support services; to include, psychosocial and nutritional programs in cancer prevention and education. A similar feasability study and planning effort is underway between The Central Vermont Hospital and MCHV so that there is a realistic goal of having a network of regionalized community cancer centers working in close cooperation with the University Center and each other to bring the best cancer management to the people of Vermont.

Vermont is a rural and mountainous state with geographic barriers of distance and poor roads coupled with periods of weather hazards which separate many cancer patients from the resources of The Vermont Regional Cancer Center. The GMOG – CCOP has provided the grass roots incentive to organize our meager resources into a regional cooperative program in cancer control.

Supported by grant CA 35091 from The National Cancer Institute, a grant from The American Cancer Society, Vermont Division, and The Green Mountain Oncology Research and Education Foundation.

Advances in Cancer Control: The War on Cancer—
15 Years of Progress, pages 217–224
© 1987 Alan R. Liss, Inc.

THE MANAGEMENT OF BREAST CANCER IN A COMMUNITY: THE IMPACT
OF THE CCOP IN FRESNO, CALIFORNIA

DeAnn Lazovich, Phyllis Ager Mowry, Marshall S.
Flam, John A. Reinsch, Debbie Butler

San Joaquin Valley Community Clinical Oncology
Program, Fresno, California, 93715

INTRODUCTION

The San Joaquin Valley Community Clinical Oncology
Program (SJV CCOP) was funded by the National Cancer
Institute (NCI) in September 1983. The NCI established the
CCOP program to bring the latest cancer therapies to the
community through clinical research. The CCOP combined
community oncologists with the large cancer population
unable or unwilling to travel to major research centers for
treatment. By encouraging oncologists to enroll patients
into protocols, patient accrual would increase, thereby
expediting the answers to scientific questions concerning
the management of cancer. Overall, the program forms a
national network consistent with NCI goals to reduce cancer
morbidity and mortality.

Stretching from Merced to Bakersfield, California, the
SJV CCOP includes 24 medical and radiation oncologists, as
well as surgeons, pathologists, radiologists and urolo-
gists. Many of the oncologists had previously participated
in clinical trials through the Northern California Oncology
Group (NCOG) and the Radiation Therapy Oncology Group
(RTOG). As part of the CCOP program, new research base
affiliations were established with the Gastrointestinal
Tumor Study Group (GITSG) and the National Surgical Adjuvant Project for Breast and Bowel Cancers (NSABP). Nearly
150 patients have been entered into various protocols each
year since the CCOP program began, with accrual to NCOG and
RTOG protocols accounting for 80% of the patients entered.

This study was undertaken to evaluate the impact of the CCOP program in the community. To accomplish this task, the discussion will center on the SJV CCOP's experience with the NSABP in Fresno County. The NSABP was selected as a model to assess community impact because it represents a new affiliation for Fresno oncologists, in which accrual doubled from 1984 to 1985, and because it focuses on breast cancer, a major disease site with considerable controversy regarding its management. An attempt will be made to evaluate whether the treatment decision for non-protocol patients seen by SJV CCOP physicians has been affected by the introduction of the CCOP program to the Fresno community.

From a historical perspective, other variables may have affected breast cancer management in this community. The passage of "The Breast Cancer Informed Consent Law" in 1980 was a major influence on the treatment of breast cancer in the State of California. It requires that women receive a "...standardized written summary...in layman's language... ..of alternative efficacious methods of treatment...when the patient is being treated for any form of breast cancer" (SB 1893, 1980). A pamphlet was published in July 1983, describing the advantages and disadvantages of alternative therapies--mastectomy (radical, modified, simple and segmental), radiotherapy and chemotherapy (California State Department of Health Services, 1983). It urges women to make an informed choice to increase personal control over a frightening disease. Although surgeons are now required by law to present the alternatives, no data is available to evaluate statewide compliance.

The publication of the results of NSABP B-06, comparing mastectomy to segmental mastectomy with or without radiation, may also have influenced the treatment decision of women diagnosed with breast cancer. The study, which appeared in the New England Journal of Medicine in March 1985, concluded that there was no difference in survival of patients managed with segmental mastectomy plus irradiation when compared to mastectomy alone (Fisher, et al, 1985). The national publicity surrounding the results may account for a change in the number of women choosing conservative or radical surgery for breast cancer. With this background, a review of the management of breast cancer in Fresno County will be conducted to determine how the SJV CCOP's participation in the NSABP has influenced the medical community.

METHODS

To measure the impact of the NSABP in Fresno County, the CCOP patient log and hospital tumor registry abstracts from two hospitals (representing 85% of the breast cancer cases in Fresno County), were analyzed for the years 1983, 1984, and 1985. The CCOP patient log is an NCI requirement to record protocol availability and treatment disposition for newly diagnosed cancer patients seen by CCOP physicians. A hospital registry with an American College of Surgeons approved Cancer Program is required to record and follow new cancer patients diagnosed at its institution for treatment and survival.

The treatment of breast cancer cases from the CCOP patient log and the hospital registries was analyzed using the CCOP log definition for adjuvant therapy decisions-- i.e., no treatment given; entered on a CCOP-approved protocol; treated on equivalent or modified arm of a CCOP-approved protocol; or other treatment regimen given. The treatment information was already available on the CCOP patient log for breast cases, but was gathered retrospectively for the registry breast cancer cases. To determine if registry patients for whom an NSABP protocol was available (based on receptor and nodal status) were treated according to an NSABP study, the chemotherapy listed in the registry abstract was compared to the treatment prescribed by the NSABP studies B-11, B-12, B-13, B-14, B-15, B-16, depending on the month and year the studies were available (Table 1). No attempt was made to eliminate ineligible protocol patients found in the registries, because the impact of the NSABP would still apply if ineligible patients were treated equivalent to an NSABP protocol. As further indication of the impact of changing medical practice on the medical community, the type of surgery, and the number of women receiving adjuvant therapy was analyzed.

Table 1. Adjuvant Breast Protocols - NSABP.

B-11: L-PAM/5FU + Adriamycin (closed 9/30/84).
B-12: L-PAM/5FU/Tamoxifen + Adriamycin (closed 9/30/84).
B-13: Methotrexate/5FU vs. No Treatment.
B-14: Tamoxifen vs. Placebo.
B-15: Adriamycin/Cytoxan (opened 10/1/84) vs.

<pre>
          Adriamycin/Cytoxan-----Rest-----CMF vs.
          CMF
B-16:   Tamoxifen (opened 10/1/84) vs.
          L-PAM/5FU/Tamoxifen/Adriamycin vs.
          Adriamycin/Cytoxan/Tamoxifen
</pre>

Both systems for registering patients have their limitations. The 1984 CCOP patient log reflects a learning process and is partially incomplete. Appropriate patients may have been missed or incorrectly logged. Registry cases may appear in more than one registry. Since registry information is gathered on an annual basis, it is possible that patients listed as receiving no subsequent therapy actually did. To reduce the chance for error, registry data was crosschecked against each other for duplication, and against the CCOP patient log for subsequent therapy missed by the registry. The registry data is complete through June of 1985; the CCOP patient log is complete through November 1985.

RESULTS

The results illustrate three distinct aspects of breast cancer therapy in the Fresno community. The first aspect is the surgical management and subsequent referral of women with a diagnosis of breast cancer. The second aspect is the potential impact of the SJV CCOP in the broad community. And the third aspect reflects the adjuvant treatment choices made by participating SJV CCOP physicians when women are referred for therapy.

In Fresno, the surgical treatment choice remains the mastectomy. Table 2 shows no significant change in the percentage of women electing segmental mastectomies from 1983 to 1985. From a total of 440 women, only 51 or 12% had this procedure. The percentage even declined in 1984, one year after the State of California published the breast pamphlet, and three years after passage of the "Informed Breast Cancer Consent Law." The information in Table 2 calls into serious question the effect of the law, the personal bias of the surgeon, and/or the treatment preference of women diagnosed with breast cancer.

TABLE 2. Type of Surgery

	MASTECTOMY	SEGMENTAL/RT	TOTAL
1983	138 (87%)	20 (13%)	158 (100%)
1984	169 (90%)	18 (10%)	187 (100%)
1985	82 (86%)	13 (14%)	95 (100%)
(6 mos.)			
TOTAL	389 (88%)	51 (12%)	440 (100%)

Important data which should direct future SJV CCOP educational efforts is seen in Table 3, indicating the number of patients receiving adjuvant therapy. The number of node-positive women undergoing treatment increased from 52% in 1983 to 83% 1985. But the category of node-negative women showed only a slight increase in the same time interval, from 8% in 1983 to 13% in 1985. It is not known whether these women with an 83-96% 5-year survival (depending on stage) were presented treatment options by their physician and elected no treatment, or if the recommendation for no further treatment was made by the physician.

TABLE 3. Number of Patients Receiving Adjuvant Therapy.

	NODE −	NODE +	TOTAL PTS TREATED
1983	9/112 (8%)	24/46 (52%)	33/158 (21%)
1984	20/128 (16%)	39/59 (66%)	59/187 (32%)
1985	7/55 (13%)	33/40 (83%)	40/95 (42%)
(6 mos.)			
TOTAL	36/295 (12%)	96/145 (66%)	132/440 (30%)

From the total number of breast cancer registry cases, the percent of patients for whom an NSABP protocol was available is 72% (158/221) in 1983, 77% (187/242) in 1984, and 84% (95/113) in 1985. The registry data shows a positive trend with increasing numbers of patients either treated on an NSABP protocol or according to protocol (Table 4). The total percentage of breast cancer patients affected by the SJV CCOP in Fresno increased from 3% in 1983, to 14% in 1984 and 25% in 1985 (first 6 months). Only 45% of the patients enrolled on NSABP studies are represented in the registries which account for most of the breast cancer diagnosed in Fresno County. Therefore the impact of the NSABP participation is likely to be greater than that shown in Table 4, if all the patients were counted.

TABLE 4. Adjuvant Treatment of Breast Cancer in the
          Community Based on Tumor Registries.

	1983		1984		1985 (6 mo.)	
	#	%	#	%	#	%
Total # Pts NSABP Protocol Available	158	100%	187	100%	95	100%
Pts Entered	1	1%	3	2%	9	9%
Modified Protocol	3	2%	22	12%	15	16%
No Treatment	117	74%	125	66%	53	56%
Other	37	23%	37	20%	18	19%

SJV CCOP physicians are actively entering patients on
NSABP studies. The experience gained from this affiliation
has influenced the treatment of many more women. Table 5
illustrates clearly the agreement in the SJV CCOP to treat
according to NSABP. Of the patients available for NSABP
protocols, 10% were entered in 1984 and 15% in 1985. When
the non-protocol patients treated according to protocol are
added, the total impact is 35% and 51% in 1984 and 1985
respectively. This represents a major finding, especially
when compared to the SJV CCOP patient log for all sites,
which only shows 22% of patients entered on protocol or
treated equivalently. Table 6 further emphasizes the
influence of NSABP on treatment decisions. The treatment
offered by SJV CCOP physicians which was influenced by the
NSABP, affected twice as many patients within the SJV CCOP
as patients in the community at large for both 1984 and
1985.

TABLE 5. Adjuvant Treatment of Breast Cancer by SJV CCOP
          Physicians (Based on CCOP Patient Log).

	BREAST						ALL SITES	
	1983		1984		1985		5/84-5/85	
	#	%	#	%	#	%	#	%
Total # Pts NSABP Protocol Available	--	--	87	100%	121	100%	629	100%
Pts Entered	2	Unkn.	9	10%	18	15%	71	11%
Modified Protocol	--	--	22	25%	44	36%	67	11%
No Treatment	--	--	20	23%	25	21%	45	7%
Other	--	--	36	41%	34	28%	350	57%
Unknown	--	--	--	--	--	--	97	15%

TABLE 6. Measurement of Impact - % Patients on Protocol or
          Modified Protocol.

	REGISTRIES	PT LOG - BREAST
1983	3%	--
1984	14%	35%
1985*	25%	51%

*6 months - Registry
11 months - Patient Log

DISCUSSION

It is rewarding to conduct an analysis which shows a
positive trend of the impact of community research, and at
the same time, points to future directions for improvement.
To better understand the results in Fresno County and the
SJV CCOP, it is useful to look at the Eastern Cooperative
Study Group (ECOG) experience. The ECOG conducted a survey
to measure the impact of cooperative groups on cancer
therapy in community hospitals (Begg, et al, 1983). Table
7 summarizes the results for ECOG community affiliates. It
shows that 9% of patients were on an ECOG protocol and 7%
were on a non-ECOG protocol. Non-protocol treatment influenced by a clinical trial was 35%, which included both ECOG
and other cooperative group studies. Added together, ECOG
determined that the measurement of impact on the community
was 51%. If the SJV CCOP results in Table 6 are compared
to the ECOG evaluation, then the NSABP influence in
Fresno's oncology community in 1985 is even stronger,
because 15% of SJV CCOP patients were entered on NSABP
(compared to 9% on ECOG studies), and the treatment disposition for another 36% was determined by NSABP alone. In
other words, more than half of the breast cancer patients
seen by SJV CCOP physicians benefitted from the NSABP
participation.

Table 7. Summary of ECOG Results.

On ECOG Protocol	9%
On IRB Protocol other than ECOG	7%
Influenced by a Protocol but not on (ECOG or other)	35%
TOTAL	51%

Clearly, the State law has not yet been effective in
Fresno, and it is too soon to evaluate the effect of the
published NSABP results on surgical management of breast
cancer. To date, only 12% of women (440 cases total) have

opted for segmental mastectomy plus irradiation. Yet, based on NSABP B-06, women have a choice of equally effective therapies. The frequency of the pamphlet distribution, the degree of physician bias in the presentation of alteratives, and the reasons for a woman's choice are not known. Further study is indicated and increased SJV CCOP efforts to heighten public and physician awareness of the NSABP data are needed. Encouraging surgeons to refer all patients for oncology evaluation and protocol participation could effectively increase accrual and contribute significantly to current knowledge about breast cancer therapy, especially for node-negative patients.

Without a doubt, the SJV CCOP has been an important force in this community to date, especially in the management of breast cancer. Attendance at NSABP meetings, distribution of information, such as the NIH Consensus Statement on breast cancer, and the development of protocol aids to facilitate protocol determination, have encouraged active SJV CCOP physician participation. With nearly every Fresno oncologist now participating in the NSABP and with the increasing accrual into NSABP protocols, the dedication of the SJV CCOP physicians to clinical research in the community is evident. The NCI objective for the CCOP program to bring current cancer therapies to the community is being realized in the San Joaquin Valley.

REFERENCES

SB 1893, 1980, Chapter 916, Section 1704.5, CA Health and Safety Code.

California State Department of Health Services, (July 1983). Breast cancer treatment summary of alternative effective methods, risks, advantages, disadvantages.

Fisher B, Bauer M, et al (1985). Five-year results of a randomized clinical trial comparing total mastectomy and segmental mastectomy with or without radiation in the treatment of breast cancer. New England J of Medicine, 312:665-673.

Begg C, Zelen M, et al (1983). Cooperative groups and community hospitals. Measurement of impact in the community hospitals. Cancer 52: (9) 1760-1767.

Advances in Cancer Control: The War on Cancer—
15 Years of Progress, pages 225–227
© 1987 Alan R. Liss, Inc.

IMPACT OF A COMPETITIVE HEALTH CARE ENVIRONMENT ON THE
VIABILITY OF MULTI HOSPITAL CANCER CONTROL PROGRAMS: 1986
AND BEYOND

Peter A. Levine, MPH, Greater Flint Area Hospital
Assembly's CHOP, 702 S. Ballenger Hwy., Flint, MI
48504, and Willys Mueller, M.D., Director of
Pathology, Hurley Medical Center, One Hurley Plaza,
Flint, MI 48502.

Most, if not all, of the multi hospital cancer control
programs cuurently in existence, were established in the
late 1970s and very early 1980s during a period of relative
institutional affluence most readily aided by an across the
board "cost plus reimbursement system." During that time,
hospitals and their physician staffs were capable of creating
an environment of constant improvement in the quality of care,
technology acquistion, and organizational risk taking, based
on the fact that if a project did not work, the cost of that
failure could be charged back to third party payers. In the
final analysis, that six or seven year period may have been
the golden age of organized regional community based oncology.
Several multi hospital oncology systems were developed during
that period of time, most of them using federal seed money.
They were designated community oncology programs or community
hospital oncology programs. The purpose of those programs
was to create a region wide improvement in quality of care,
through standardization. This was to be achieved through
the development of regional treatment guidelines.

In addition, several programs including the non federally
funded Flint area CHOP, achieved increased physician interest
in clinical research, educational programming, and outreach,
both in terms of screening and direct patient accrual through
external marketing. Programs such as the Flint CHOP have
been able to standardize care at an elevated level and income
for its member institutions. Those hospitals include: 1980-
1985 St. Joseph Hospital; 1980-1986 Hurley Medical Center,
Flint Osteopathic Hospital, McLaren General Hospital, Wheelock
Hospital, and Lapeer General Hospital.

With the advent of prospective payment systems, many cooperative cancer programs have begun to fall by the wayside, due to the fact that key physicians or institutions perceive the need to become more insular. This leads to a competitive strategy rather than one of cooperation. In addition, for several consortia or systems, simply attracting more patients through cooperation did not lead to the proper mix of resource expenditure versus resources accrued. As a consequence, some communities experienced a diminution in participation in multi hospital cancer control programs, leading to a perception of benefit to the institutions not remaining equal to or greater than the costs.

In the greater Flint area, the non federally funded CHOP has been better positioned to accommodate the program costs than have several governmentally funded programs, due to the fact that the hospitals were never traumatized by withdrawal of governmental funding in the regional cancer control programs. There never has been any. Although one hospital has left the program, it has not, as of this date, entered into the realm of open competition against the membership of the CHOP. The program has remained viable financially, unlike many of the programs across the nation both larger and smaller. The goals and objectives of the Greater Flint Area Hospital Assembly's CHOP have shifted quite substantially over the course of its five and a half years of existence. Due to the fact that qualitative aspects of the program are in place and ongoing, the goal shift has moved to the area of promotion of member institutions and their physicians through education rather than through advertisement. It would appear that many programs across the country are still operating according to the original program goals and objectives which basically involve assuring cooperation between institutions and reducing outflow of patients. The Flint CHOP provides on-site educational programming for physicians and institutions on a statewide basis, both through traditional methods and through live teleconferencing on key cancer control issues.

Financing methods for multi hospital cancer control programs continue to run the gamut from being: wholly federally funded; partially federally funded with some foundation or hospital support; or totally hospital or foundation supported. While this has not altered in terms of the broad scope, individual programs have been involved in transitions. Many of the federally funded programs which have not gone out

of existence, are now privately funded, either by the health
care industry locally or by foundations. The CCOPs have
brought new monies into several communities which have not
previously attracted federal monies. It is anticipated,
however, that following the recompetition of the CCOPs, that
many programs will be forced to seek private funding while
programs as the Flint CHOP which has historically had six
hospital members paying proportionate dues remain relatively
stable.

The level of physician support for regional cancer control
activities is probably the key to maintaining a multi hospital
cancer control program. Those cancer programs which are not
able to maintain the interest in each hospital's key cancer
related physician will rapidly find institutional membership
shrinkage. It appears that over-all physician participation
peaks after three years of operations and then tails off to
a support level of only key cancer practitioners. Interestingly
enough, the Flint experience has shown significantly increases
in the participation of general and family practitioners
through years four and five. This has been due to the fact
that those physicians have been targeted for participation
through various activities such as screening and education.

Finally, a trend is developing for hospitals to hire
highly skilled administrators to manage their individual
oncology rpograms and for consortia to hire trained administrators or medical care organization sepecialists to manage
multi hospital oncology programs. In addition, multi hospital
corporations are beginning to incorporate staff with strong
administrative skills, to assure the growth of oncology within
their pervue. High technology acquisitions, as well as research protocol involvement is more highly scrutinized now
than ever before, due to cost involvement. The involvement
of key physicians in the management decision making process
is also becoming evermore common; a development which is
expected to lead to a more pervasive integration of the administrative and medical decision making process.

The multi hospital cancer control program appears to be
a concept which is slipping in terms of popularity, but which
is needed more now than before. The diminution of competition
between institutions is a more cost beneficial route to follow,
than is that of open and extremely costly inter-hospital blood
letting in a resource intensive field such as oncology.

Advances in Cancer Control: The War on Cancer—
15 Years of Progress, pages 229-232
© 1987 Alan R. Liss, Inc.

THE IMPORTANCE OF MULTI HOSPITAL LINKAGES FOR ONCOLOGICAL
CANCER CONTROL SERVICES TO THE RURAL HOSPITAL: AN ADMINI-
STRATIVE PERSPECTIVE

Peter A. Levine, MPH, Greater Flint Area Hospital
Assembly's CHOP, 702 S. Ballenger Hwy., Flint,
MI 48504, and Isak Berker, M.D., Lapeer General
Hospital, 1375 N. Main St., Lapeer, MI 48446

The 1980's will be remembered as a decade of intense
competition in the hospital industry. This competitive
environment is causing some multi hospital oncology and
cancer control programs to lose part or all of their membership and as a consequence to lose part or all of their funding. In addition, the developing insular nature of individual
hospitals and of the independent physician practices are
resulting in moves to reduce outreach or cooperation between
institutions, especially between urban and rural hospitals.
This is increasingly due to the lack of trust of the larger
urban hospitals by the smaller rural hospitals. This insular
stance occurs at a time when cancer care services are becoming
more sophisticated with expanded technological and staffing
requirements. These staffing and capitol intensive requirements can easily be beyond the scope of that which a rural
hospital board of trustees can support. At the same time,
pressure exists to advance the standards of practice in
oncology. This pressure leads to an ever increasing need
to provide the broad spectrum of cancer care services
regardless of the locale of the institution or physician
practice.

The authors propose that there is a broad spectrum of
activities which rural hospitals may implement to affilate
with larger institutions, which will result in the rural
hospital's ability to provide a broader scope of cancer
services, to the benefit of both institutions and to the
patients. These actions will lead to: a reduction of out-
of-region referrals from the rural and urban community
hospitals; an increase in rural patient utilization of urban

hospitals; an improved quality of care for rural patients; increased rural area physician income due to the control of the flow of the patient's care by the attending physician; and access to a new patient population of research and specialized diagnostic and therapeutic services available at the larger affiliate institution.

Probably the primary reason for reticence on the part of rural institutions to affiliate with major urban institutions is the fact that the urban institution will often retain the rural patient for therapy beyond the period required to perform complex or advanced therapeutic or diagnostic services. An urban institution must realize that rural institutions know what is occurring and are capable of tracking patient activity through newly implemented computerized patient information systems available at most hospitals.

Should a rural institution decide to approach an urban institution regarding the provision of advanced or research procedures, it is imperative that the rural institution clarify the role that the urban institution is expected to play. With the environment requiring increased admissions, reduced lengths of stay, and increased utilization of out-patient services, all institutions can benefit from the effectively monitored transfers back and forth of patients from urban to rural and rural to urban institutions. The net result will be that all participants in this system benefit, including the patient, the hospital, and physician.

Very few rural institutions have ready access to medical and surgical residents and interns, yet many would be willing to participate in a training in cooperation with an urban hospital. The benefit of access to that type of personnel is clearly evident to a rural institution. The benefit to the urban institution with a residency or internship program, is not always so clear. In addition, the evidence of benefit to the intern or resident may be less intrinsically clear. The point must be made that the provision of a rural hospital experience to an intern or resident, the great merit from all three perspectives. There is no question, that the majority of positions available for graduating or newly trained physicians, are in the rural areas. Learning about rural environments and the rural health care system will provide the intern or resident with a readily available source of experiential data gathering. It is also a service which an urban hospital can provide to a rural hospital to show good faith in the exchange of services and patients, required to maintain a good working relationship with effective transfer agreements.

Referrals by rural physicians to large urban institution as a referral locale, due to the fact that the closer the urban institution, the less likely it is to be perceived as "expert." In addition, physicians often do not wish to send their "problem cases" to a locale close enough to involve risk to their reputation. The patient is also likely to perceive an institution which is further away to be more expert. This traditional referral pattern, results in significant lost income to the local rural institution, the nearby urban institutions, and the attending and specialist physician population in both the rural and urban communities. Explanation of the situation and its income ramifications to rural and urban physicians can result in a significant change in referral patterns.

The development of an affiliation agreement with an urban hospital, can enhance the reputation of the rural hospital, in the community that it serves. This has obvious positive financial and reputational benefits and can be aggressively pursued.

Through effective management of interactions between hospitals, and medical staffs, incorporating the suggestions listed above, with those cancer control projects established by the Greater Flint Area Hospital Assembly's CHOP, dramatic results can be achieved. Referrals to out-of-region hospitals can be slashed to insignificant levels and substantial increased revenues generated by all parties.

A recent CHOP study demonstrates results achieved among the hospitals participating in the Greater Flint Area Hospital Assembly's CHOP: Hurley Medical Center, Flint Osteopathic Hospital, McLaren General Hospital, Wheelcok Memorial Hospital, St. Joseph Hospital, and Lapeer General Hospital. Two of the member hospitals are rural and four urban. The cooperative system established in the fourth quarter of 1980 has reaped substantial benefits to the participating physicians and institutions, and provided significant improvements in access for all of the residents of Genesee, Lapeer, and Shiawassee Counties. Noteworthy on this chart, is a reduction of 6,839 cancer patient days referred to out-of-region hospitals, and an inflow increase of 259 cancer patient days in the third year of operations, 1983. To determine the revenues accrued, think in terms of 6,839 patient days X (times) average regional inpatient charge per day, and one can determine the potential benefit to an institution or set of institutions, in terms of inpatient revenue alone. Outpatient and physician office revenues were not tested.

Also noteworthy is the site specific data. It denotes the need to work closely with members of subspecialty groups from the start, evidencing cooperation between institutions and practices, to achieve greater compliance with referrals as per the agreements between hospitals to achieve the desired outcome.

Advances in Cancer Control: The War on Cancer—
15 Years of Progress, pages 233–236
© 1987 Alan R. Liss, Inc.

THE IMPACT ON REDUCING REFERRALS OF CANCER PATIENTS TO OUT-
OF-REGION HOSPITALS RESULTING FROM THE IMPLEMENTATION OF A
MULTI HOSPITAL REGIONAL CANCER CONTROL PROGRAM

Peter A. Levine, MPH, Greater Flint Area Hospital
Assembly's CHOP, 702 S. Ballenger Hwy., Flint, MI
48504 and Dan George, MPA, Hurley Medical Center,
One Hurley Plaza, Flint, MI 48502

A recently completed Community Wide Hospital Oncology
Program Patient Origin Study has dramatically demonstrated
the impact of the CHOP process on patterns of care in the
Genesee, Lapeer, and Shiawassee County HSA region of Michigan.
The CHOP study evaluated cancer patient influx from outside
of the GLS region; GLS cancer patient fow to out-of-region
hospitals; and GLS area cancer patients cared for in the GLS
area hospitals. The study utilized 1980, and compared that
data to that of 1983.

A brief synopsis of the data shows that cancer patient
admissions increased in the GLS region during that period by
17%, during a period of time in which overall GLS area medical
and surgical admissions dropped by 6.5%. The data shows that
although there was an 8% drop in inpatient medical and surgical
days across the board from 1980 to 1983 in the greater Flint
area, CHOP member hospitals experienced only a 1/10 of a
day reduction per cancer patient admission in terms of length
of stay. In addition, the data shows the outflow of GLS area
patients to Detroit, Ann Arbor, and Lansing hospitals was
reduced by 73.4%, as well as by 75.9% in terms of patient days.
Finally, the influx of cancer patient days from outside of
the region increased by 6.57% during that period of time.
The number of cancer patients attracted to GLS region hospitals
increased by 10.94%.

The data validates the CHOP process, at least the fashion
in which it was implemented in the greater Flint area. Through
a multi hospital and physician practice effort, state-of-the-art
care has been available to a broad spectrum of patients, and

the need to ship large numbers of patients to major centers
has been alleviated.

The body site specific data is also quite dramatic. The
data demonstrates the positive impact in terms of increased
recoupment of patients for which guidelines were developed.
This further validates the CHOP process indicating that the
communication patterns developed through the CHOP have made
more physicians aware of what is available within the greater
Flint area in terms of cancer care, thus reducing the perceived
need to refer patients to out-of-region institutions.

The establishment of the guidelines has also eliminated,
up until this point in time, the liability risks of providing
cancer care. Only one cancer related malpractice case has
been filed since the standards were developed, and the case
was dismissed.

The data shows that:

- In 1980, a total of 3,136 cancer patients were treated
  in the greater Flint area. In 1983, that number increased by 534 to 3,670. This represents a 17% increase
  of cancer patient admissions.

- The outflow of GLS area cancer patients to Detroit,
  Ann Arbor, and Lansing hospitals in 1980 was 631.
  In 1983, that number was reduced by 463 to 168 patients.
  This represents a reduction in out referrals of 73.4%.

- Patient influx comparisons between 1980 and 1983 show
  that in 1983, 265 cancer patients were attracted to
  the Flint area hospitals from outside of the GLS region.
  In 1983, 294 cancer patients were attracted to the GLS
  region hospitals, representing an increase of 29 patients
  or 10.94%.

- In 1980, cancer patient days treated in the CHOP member
  hospitals numbered 47,966. That number increased by
  15.3% in 1983, to 55,322.

- The outflow of cancer patient days to southeastern
  Michigan and South Central Michigan in 1980 represented
  9.008 patient days. In 1983, the outflow of patient
  days was 2,169, a reduction of 6,839 days or 75.9%.

- The influx of cancer patient days show an increase from 3,940 patient days, to 4,199 patient days.

The review of site specific figures is of significant interest. The numbers include, do not forget, a 1980 baseline and a comparison year of 1983.

FOR TREATMENT OF CANCER OF THE LIP AND ORAL CAVITY

The outflow of patient days was cut 70.59%. This represents a recoupment of 401 days; total patients treated in the region for lip and oral cancer increased by 92.1%; total patient days resulting from cancers of the lip and oral cavity increased by 171.47%, from 333 days in 1980 to 904 patient days in 1983.

FOR COLON CANCER

The number of patients treated in the region on an inpatient basis increased by 48.58%, from 177 to 263; days for colon cancer increased by 43.19%, from 3,329 to 4,767; this is an increase of 1,438 days in three years; the outflow of patients to out-of-region hospitals dropped by 92.3%; the outflow of inpatient days was decreased by 93.98%; that figure represents a recouping of 469 days; inflow of patients was increased by 85.71%; inflow of days increased by 71.74%.

FOR CANCERS OF THE BRONCHUS, LUNG AND TRACHEA

The number of patients treated increased by 17.2%; the outflow of patients was cut by 78%; the outflow of patient days was decreased by 81%, representing the recoupment of 1,180 patient days; 1,180 patient days represents approximately $590,000 recouped.

FOR BREAST CANCER

The outflow of patients was cut by 90.32%, which resulted in an elimination of 93.63% of the days which were shipped to out-of-region hospitals in 1980.

FOR CANCERS OF THE BRAIN

The total number of brain cancer patients increased between 1980 and 1983 by 92.85%. Total days increased by 161.04% or 897 days. The outflow of patients was cut by 80% and days by 74.4%. The increase in days of 897 represents approximately $44,500 in recouped revenue.

FOR GU CANCERS

The most dramatic changes took place in the GU cancers. For bladder cancer out referrals decreased by 92.85%, while out referred days were cut by 97.67%. For prostate cancer, out referrals were cut by 100%, as were out referred days, a recoupment of 317 days. In referrals increased by 10.53% and days by 28.51%.

Overall figures for hematology were as good as those for solid tumors.

In essence, cost of the CHOP in hospital dues for 1980 through 1983 was less than $100,000 while the recouping of 7,000 patient days in 1983 alone generated the member institutions $4,045,800 in inpatient revenue. Physician fees, outpatient services and other services were probably equal to another several million dollars.

Advances in Cancer Control: The War on Cancer—
15 Years of Progress, pages 237–242
© 1987 Alan R. Liss, Inc.

LIFE AFTER CHOP: WHEN A COMMUNITY CARES ABOUT CANCER CARE

Donna J. Stover, R.N., B.S.N.

Administrative Director, Kalamazoo Community
Hospital Oncology Program, 1521 Gull Road,
Kalamazoo, Michigan 49001

An appropriate subtitle for this paper might be, "Yes,
Virginia, There Can Be A CHOP Program After The Federal
Dollars Are Gone." This paper will discuss the Kalamazoo
Community Hospital Oncology Program (KCHOP) during the
National Cancer Institute (NCI) years, describe the overall
plans for continuing the program and funding the program,
and lastly describe plans to assure the future health of
the program.

The KCHOP is a consortium of Bronson Methodist Hospital
and Borgess Medical Center, two 450 bed acute care hospitals
located in Kalamazoo, Michigan. At the time of the CHOP
Request for Proposal (RFP), each hospital had a fairly well
developed cancer program with tumor registries, dedicated
inpatient units, outpatient cancer clinics, medical
oncologists, radiation oncologists, and satellite
affiliation with the Eastern Cooperative Oncology Group
(ECOG) through Rush Presbyterian/St. Luke's. The two
hospitals serve a nine county area in Southwest Michigan
with a population of over 800,000 people.

Like most hospitals located near one another, there was
intense rivalry between Borgess and Bronson in most areas
and there still is. However, cancer care is no longer a
cause for fierce rivalry. A spirit of cooperation and
collaboration reigns over the joint cancer program. The
American College of Surgeons surveyed and granted three
year joint approval to the KCHOP last spring as a community
program.

Like many other communities and hospitals, Kalamazoo applied for and was awarded a CHOP contract. The program was developed under the NCI umbrella. These federal dollars provided the seed money, as they did in many other areas of the country, for a well organized community cancer program. The following chart outlines the organization of the program. (See Table 1).

During the NCI years of funding, the KCHOP contributed to improved care and monitoring of care by developing the following:

-- computerized data management system
-- site specific cancer care guidelines
-- nursing care plans
-- rehabilitation and continuing care system
-- Community Clinical Oncology Program (CCOP)
-- American College of Surgeons approval for each hospital
-- plan for continued funding

For the continuation of the program, the last accomplishment has been the most important. By planning ahead, some of the classic pitfalls of programs started, completed, and ended under federal dollars have been avoided. This planning started with the NCI application. A plan for community support of the KCHOP after the soft money was gone was written into the original response to the RFP.

The plan called for the creation of a consortium committee. This committee includes the following individuals: two members from each hospital Board of Trustees, Chief of Staff from each hospital, Vice Chief of Staff from each hospital, one key hospital administrator from each hospital, program's Medical Director, and the program's Administrative Director. The committee is the equivalent of a Board of Directors to the program. This group has been responsible for supervision and planning for the entire program, communication with medical staffs, Boards of Trustees, and administrations, budget approval, and program funding.

Early in the programmatic development of the KCHOP the Consortium Committee elected to create an endowment program to ensure the continuation of the program after

Figure 1

ORGANIZATIONAL STRUCTURE

Kalamazoo Community Hospital Oncology Program

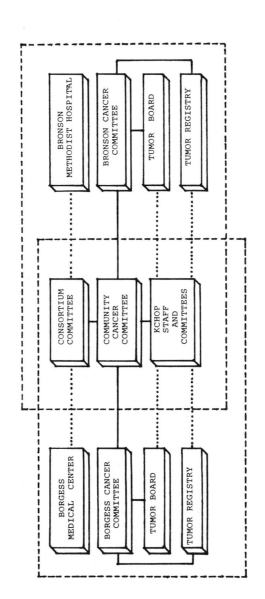

federal dollars ceased. The Kalamazoo Foundation was asked
to manage this endowment. The Foundation invests and
manages the endowment monies, invoices pledges, and gives
the program local credibility.

The major seed for the endowment came from the
Kalamazoo Academy of Medicine. It was the beneficiary of a
will which the benefactor had restricted for the creation
of a cancer registry for Kalamazoo. Local lay community
leaders were recruited to assist with fund raising. Emphasis
was shifted to include these individuals as an integral
part of the program. A prominent businessman and a retired
bank president were asked to co-chair the fund raising
efforts. Together they created a three phase program. (See
Table 2).

Phase I was the first year without federal dollars. To
allow the program time to build the necessary endowment,
the two hospitals agreed to each fund 50 percent of the
program with the understanding that their contributions
would begin to decrease in subsequent years. Phase II
encompasses a three year period of time and was planned to
be the period of active fund raising and endowment growth.
Phase III will begin when the endowment goal has been
realized and interest income can support one-third of the
program's financial needs.

The program is now in the second year of Phase II of
the funding plan. The co-chairs of the fund raising effort
are utilizing letters followed by personal visits. Phase II
funding sources include physicians, local business and
industry, key citizens, and memorial contributions. A short
slide presentation is available, a brochure describing the
program has been developed and can be included in mailings
or used with a personal visit. Pledge envelopes and
memorial gift envelopes have been printed and are being
used. Besides the two co-chairs, a group of ten physicians
have been recruited to help with contacting their colleagues
for funds. We have developed and prioritized several
categorized lists for funding sources.

Throughout this time, it has been important to maintain
a balanced, highly visible, meaningful program. As hospital
competition remits and exacerbates, the program must always
remain neutral. Furthermore, it is critical to the program
to maintain both its own identity and some degree of

Figure 2

THREE PHASE FUNDING PROGRAM

	1984/85	1985/86	1986/87	1987/88	1988/89	1989 & BEYOND
P H A S E I	50% BORGESS 50% BRONSON ───── 100%	35% BORGESS 35% BRONSON 30% FOUNDATIONS ───── 100%	35% BORGESS 35% BRONSON 30% FOUNDATIONS ───── 100%	35% BORGESS 35% BRONSON 30% FOUNDATIONS ───── 100%	33.3% BORGESS 33.3% BRONSON 0 FOUNDATIONS 33.3% INT. INCOME ───── 100%	

P H A S E II

SOLICITATION:

-Physicians
-Corporations
-Individual
 Major Gifts
-Miscellaneous
 Gifts, Pledges
 and Memorials

Endowment
Growth

↑

P H A S E III

INTEREST
INCOME:

At 8%   =33.3%
Borgess=33.3%
Bronson=33.3%
       ─────
        100%

autonomy while at the same time allowing each hospital to feel ownership of the program. Each hospital continues to be committed and involved in KCHOP. The program has to some degree provided "oil on the water" for the community as each hospital uses KCHOP to demonstrate that they can and do get along with the other hospital when it really counts.

This cooperation and continued financial support has allowed the program to continue and grow beyond the National Cancer Institute CHOP contract. Recent accomplishments include:

-- guideline update
-- nursing care plan revision
-- colorectal screening projects
-- health risk assessment for senior citizens with the Red Cross
-- collaborative professional and public education programs with community agencies
-- American College of Surgeons approval of a Community Oncology Program (3 years)

Plans for the future include continual guideline revisions, continual nursing care plan revisions, continual medical education, nursing cancer patient education program, five year survival studies, site-a-month data analysis and cancer control projects aimed at prevention and early detection.

In summary, the KCHOP has been successful during CHOP and beyond due to some key elements. First, the program planned ahead and included continuing funding as part of the RFP, the medical community and community leaders were involved in planning, implementation and continuation of the program, volunteers were used to decrease expenses, the program has been highly visible, and both hospital and community leaders have had a high degree of ownership in the program. The KCHOP plans to be a dynamic and integral part of cancer care in Kalamazoo for years to come.

CLINICAL AND EPIDEMIOLOGICAL RESEARCH IN THE COMMUNITY

Advances in Cancer Control: The War on Cancer—
15 Years of Progress, pages 245–253
© 1987 Alan R. Liss, Inc.

CANCER ETIOLOGY, MANAGEMENT, AND OUTCOME: DOES IT MATTER WHO YOU ARE?

Hari H. Dayal, Ph.D.
Epi-Stat Research Laboratory
Fox Chase Cancer Center, Philadelphia, PA and the
Dept. of Preventive Medicine and Community Health,
University of Texas Medical Branch, Galveston, TX

Etiology, diagnosis, management, compliance, and survival are some of the important elements of the continuum describing a cancer episode. The "who" may apply variously to each of these elements. For example: who gets the disease (the etiology); who is diagnosed early; who is managed optimally; who complies with the regimen; and who survives the disease. Let us restrict the "who" to two dimensions, namely, race and socioeconomic status (SES). Race and SES are highly correlated in the United States; whether the measure used for SES is education, occupation, income, or a combination of these variables, a higher proportion of Blacks than Whites are found to be at the lower end of the socioeconomic scale. Hence the relationship (correlation, association) of an outcome variable with one induces a relationship with the other. It is, therefore, difficult sometimes to discern the importance of one vis-a-vis the other.

Table 1 shows that the incidence of some cancers is related to race. Table 2 shows that socioeconomic status, either globally or through an identified component, is associated with the rates of occurrence of certain cancers. In most cases the relationship is inverse, that is, low SES populations have higher incidence; notable exceptions are cancers of the breast, colon, corpus uteri and ovary. From these two tables one would infer that who you are in terms of race and SES may have something to do with the probability of getting the disease.

TABLE 1: Race and Cancer Incidence:
Average Annual Age-Adjusted Incidence Rates
for Selected Sites per 100,000

Primary Site	White	Black
Esophagus	3.0	10.0
Stomach	8.6	15.4
Lung & Bronchus (M)	76.4	110.0
Cervix Uteri (F)	10.9	25.7
Corpus Uteri (F)	29.9	14.6
Bladder (M)	27.0	13.6
Melanoma	6.3	0.7
Multiple myeloma	3.5	7.9
Prostate gland (M)	66.2	108.9
Breast (F)	85.6	72.0

Compiled from: Surveillance, Epidemiology, End Results:
Incidence and Mortality Data, 1973-1977. National Cancer
Institute Monograph 57. June 1981.

TABLE 2: Etiologic Role of SES in
Various Cancer Sites

Site	Relationship with SES	Site	Relationship with SES
Lip, oral cavity	Inverse	Cervix Uteri	Inverse, strong
Esophagus	Inverse	Corpus Uteri	Direct
Stomach	Inverse	Ovary	Direct
Colon	Direct, weak	Prostate	Inverse
Liver	Inverse	Penis	Inverse, weak
Pancreas	Inverse	Scrotum	Inverse
Larynx	Inverse	Bladder	Inverse, related to occupation & smoking
Lung	Inverse		
Skin (excluding melanoma)	Inverse, related to occupation	Hodgkin's Disease	Direct to education, inverse to family size
Breast	Direct	Leukemia	Direct, weak

Compiled from: Cancer Risks by Site, International Union
Against Cancer, TEchnical Report Series, Volume 41, 1980.

Once the disease has been initiated, the issues of diagnosis and management become crucial. The various components are: detection (early or late), stage of the disease at diagnosis, treatments offered, compliance with the treatment regimen, support systems, and follow-up. Clearly, the mode of identification and management of the disease has an important bearing on the outcome--the cure rate and the probability of surviving a given length of time after diagnosis.

The national data (Axtell and Myers, 1978) show that, for most cancers, survival from cancer among Blacks is poorer than among Whites. These inferences are sometimes questioned because of the lack of uniformity in treatment patterns, quality control and definition of data items. But, analyses from single medical institutions also suggest that Blacks and/or low SES patients have poorer survival prognosis for most cancers. For instance, Figures 1 and 2 based on data from the Medical College of Virginia clearly showed a survival advantage for the White patients for prostate cancer and breast cancer. These data also showed a relationship between SES and survival probability (Dayal and Chiu, 1982; Dayal et al 1982). Moreover, the association between race (and SES) and survival persisted after adjustment for age and disease stage.

Figures 3 and 4 (Dayal et al, 1987) are based on a subset of data from the Centralized Cancer Patient Data System (CCPDS) representing comprehensive cancer centers with racially balanced patient populations. For both colon cancer and rectal cancer, these data showed a significant difference in survival by race. In the multivariate regression analyses of survival time, race emerged as a significant factor in predicting the probability of survival. A stage-specific multivariate analysis revealed that, for either cancer, the difference in survival between Blacks and Whites was most pronounced for patients with localized disease. This is a particularly interesting finding in view of the fact that colo-rectal cancer can be managed effectively by surgery in the localized stage.

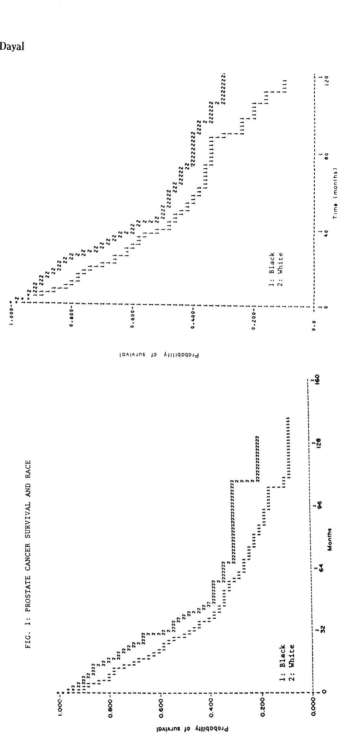

FIG. 2: BREAST CANCER SURVIVAL AND RACE

1: Black
2: White

Source: Dayal et al, J Chron Dis 35, 1982, pp 675-683

FIG. 1: PROSTATE CANCER SURVIVAL AND RACE

1: Black
2: White

Source: Dayal et al, J Chron Dis 35, 1982, pp 553-560

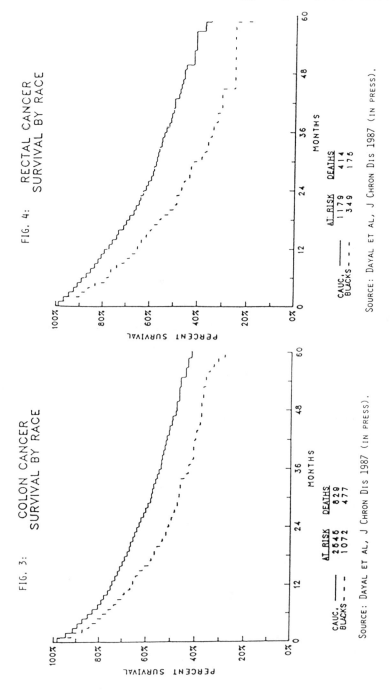

FIG. 4: RECTAL CANCER
SURVIVAL BY RACE

FIG. 3: COLON CANCER
SURVIVAL BY RACE

TABLE 3: Percent of Cancers not Treated by Primary Site

	CCPDS		NATIONAL	
	WHITES	BLACKS	WHITES	BLACKS
COLON	5.1	9.6	11	16
RECTUM	6.0	12.9	12	21
BLADDER	4.0	8.2	4	14
KIDNEY	1.5	5.6	11	15
UTERINE CORPUS	2.9	8.7	3	13
UTERINE CERVIX	8.2	10.8	5	11
BREAST	2.7	4.4	3	5

SOURCES:

National: Contrasts in Survival of Black and White Cancer
Patients, 1960-1973, by Lillian Axtell, M.A., and Max H.
Myers, Ph.D. in JNCI, Vol. 60, No. 6, June 1978, p1209-1213.

CCPDS: Statistical Analysis and Quality Control Center,
Centralized Cancer Patient Data System, 1124 Columbia St.,
Seattle, WA 98104.

Let us focus on one aspect of management--the treatment.
Table 3 shows that in the CCPDS data for comprehensive cancer
centers with racially balanced populations as well as in the
SEER data, a higher proportion of Blacks compared to Whites
did not receive a tumor-directed treatment. (The proportion
of patients not receiving any tumor-directed treatment is
lower in the comprehensive cancer center consortium compared
to the national figures.) One may justifiably argue that the
higher percentage of no-treatment among Blacks could be partly
attributed to the fact that Blacks present with advanced
disease more often. But the CCPDS data show that, for any
given stage of the disease, a higher proportion of Blacks do
not receive a tumor-directed treatment. For localized disease,
in particular, 6.8% Black compared to 2.5% White colon cancer
patients, and 10.7% Black compared to 3.3% White rectal cancer
patients did not receive a curative treatment. (These data
also suggested a trend in the proportion of no-treatment group
by SES--the higher the SES, the smaller the proportion of
untreated patients.) While the absolute percentage of localized colo-rectal cancer patients who remain untreated is small,
it is disturbing that three times as many Black as White (or,
almost three times as many low SES as high SES) patients do
not receive appropriate treatment. Moreover, from the point
of view of avoidable mortality, these statistics relate to a
disease condition that can be potentially cured.

These associations are based on tumor-registry-type secondary data and, hence, several caveats may apply. For example, what if the data on treatment are erroneous? To examine this issue, we compared the survival of localized disease patients coded as receiving no treatment with the survival of those patients who had been coded as receiving some form of cancer-related treatment. For either cancer, there was a highly significant ($p < 10^{-6}$) difference between the two groups indicating mutual corroboration of survival and treatment data in the database. One may also argue that localized disease patients receiving no treatment may have been understaged, that is, these patients may actually have had regional spread. In entertaining such an hypothesis one wonders as to why such understaging, if present, should influence the two races differently. In fact, the same argument may apply to a number of other conjectures advanced to explain the difference in treatment patterns observed in these data. Age of the patient is one of the factors con- sidered in recommending surgery for the localized disease and a difference in the age distribution of localized disease patients of the two races may partially account for the dif- ference in treatment patterns. The age distribution of localized disease patients from the two races were similar in our series; if anything, Black patients were a bit younger than Caucasians. Also, there was no difference between the two races with regard to the age distribution of patients with localized disease who received no treatment.

What are the plausible explanations and hypotheses for the observed difference in treatment patterns by race/SES and the well-documented stage specific differences in survival by race and/or SES? Of course, one may hypothesize that the biology of the disease differs by race and that is the dominant factor in racial differences in treatment and survival. If one discounts this hypothesis, however, one has to postulate a scenario involving socio-cultural and behavioral dimensions. Fig. 5 describes such a conceptual hypothesis. The race (SES) may be related to the quality of care, to the support system, and perhaps to the physical condition of the host. The util- ization of cancer services may also be a function of race or SES. Perhaps the most important link between race (SES) and survival is through the compliance with the treatment regimen-- behavioral compliance as well as medical compliance. Each of these factors, singly or in an interactive multivariate fashion, may influence the length of survival after diagnosis.

Fig. 5: A Plausible Pathway Through Which Race or SES may Influence Survival

For a Given Stage at Diagnosis:

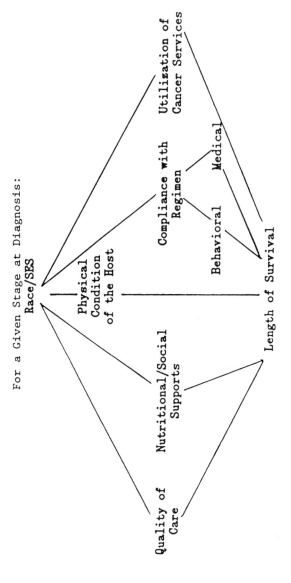

If management of the disease is an issue in explaining the racial difference in survival, what are the various micro-hypotheses in this regard? Could there be a difference in the treatment offered? Is patient-physician communication a barrier? One may also hypothesize that there is a difference in the acceptability of the treatment. A number of factors tend to support such a hypothesis a priori. For instance, differences in the perception of treatment outcomes may influence treatment acceptance. Such differences in perceptions may result from the differences in perceptions of the body image and functions, and differences in the knowledge and attitude about cancer. In reviewing charts of a limited series of patients with localized colo-rectal cancer, the common factors revealed for "no treatment" were fear of colostomy, denial of the problem, and a fatalistic attitude.

The above discussion identifies the problem, presents some secondary data, and deduces some coherent hypotheses. The importance of finding answers to these questions as far as avoidable mortality is concerned should be quite obvious. It will require a well-designed multi-institutional study representing populations of various race/SES characteristics to investigate the proposed hypotheses. Answers to these questions should then be translated into specific intervention strategies. Involvement of community hospitals is clearly the key to the proposed study and subsequent interventions. I might conclude by noting that we are in the process of initiating such a study.

REFERENCES

Axtell L, Myers M: Contrasts in survival of Black and White cancer patients, 1960-73. JNCI 60:1209-1213, 1978.

Dayal H. Chiu C: Factors associated with racial differences in survival for prostatic carcinoma. J Chron Dis 35: 553-560, 1982.

Dayal H. Power RN, and Chiu C: Race and socioeconomic status in survival from breast cancer. J Chron Dis 35:675-683, 1982.

Dayal H, Polissar L, Yang C, and Dahlberg S: Race, socio-economic status, and other prognostic factors for survival from colo-rectal cancer. J Chron Dis (in press).

Advances in Cancer Control: The War on Cancer—
15 Years of Progress, pages 255–262
© 1987 Alan R. Liss, Inc.

USE OF FOOD FREQUENCY TECHNIQUES IN EPIDEMIOLOGIC RESEARCH

R. Sue McPherson and Guy R. Newell

Department of Cancer Prevention and Control, The
University of Texas M. D. Anderson Hospital and
Tumor Institute, Houston, Texas 77030

BACKGROUND

It is estimated that by the year 2000 there will be
84,000 cases of cancer diagnosed in Texas per year as
compared to about 43,000 cases in 1983. That is almost
double the number of new cases in seventeen years. Much of
this rise in the number of cases of cancer in Texas is due
to projected increases in the number of individuals living
in Texas and to the aging of the population.

There are three major ethnic groups in Texas – Anglos,
Blacks, and Hispanics. The varied ethnic composition of
these counties provided the opportunity to compare the
incidence of several types of cancer among ethnic groups
(Table 1).

Table 1. Cancer Incidence* of Selected Sites
by Ethnic Group in Texas

Site	White		Black		Hispanic	
	M	F	M	F	M	F
Breast	–	61.6	–	45.3	–	28.7
Colon	22.8	26.0	14.3	18.7	9.0	12.2
Stomach	14.8	8.1	28.0	13.3	23.4	14.9
Lung	38.8	–	35.0	–	19.4	–

*Incidence per 100,000 age adjusted to the 1970 U.S.
male/female population (Macdonald et al, 1978).

In Texas, Black and Spanish-surnamed men have a lower incidence of lung and colon cancer and a higher incidence of cancer of the stomach than among Anglos. Black and Spanish-surnamed women in Texas have less breast and colon cancer, yet an increased incidence of stomach cancer than among Anglos. Hispanics in Texas have a 2- to 3-fold increase in the risk of cancer of the breast and colon than do Anglos (Batcher, et al, 1984).

Evidence from epidemiologic and laboratory studies suggests that dietary factors may be associated with these cancers. In fact, it has been suggested that dietary factors may be associated with up to 35% of all cancers (Bazzare, et al, 1980). One hypothesis regarding the role of diet in cancer development is that some foods contain initiating as well as direct carcinogenic components. A second hypothesis suggests that consumption or lack of consumption of specific foods establishes a condition that enhances organ susceptibility and response to other cancer causing factors. These hypotheses imply that certain foods contain nutrients which may play a preventive role in the neoplastic process (Block, 1982). A possible explanation of the differences in site specific cancer incidence in ethnic groups in Texas, is that the Hispanics and Blacks consume different foods. For example, foods indigenous to the Hispanic culture could contain more cancer-inhibiting substances or less cancer-causing substances than foods eaten by other ethnic groups (NRC, 1982).

NUTRITIONAL EPIDEMIOLOGY

Epidemiologists wishing to study this hypothesized relationship of dietary factors to cancer incidence have limited options regarding the method of ascertaining dietary information. Valid and reliable methods to measure individual dietary intake that are quick, inexpensive, and sufficiently simple to be used in large epidemiologic studies are not readily available (Doll, et al, 1981). More specifically, there are no available data concerning the reliability or validity of dietary measurement tools for classifying the intakes of different ethnic subgroups (Macdonald, et al, 1978).

The method commonly selected to ascertain diet exposure data for epidemiologic studies is the food frequency questionnaire. Food frequency questionnaires consist of a list of foods and a set of frequency response options to indicate how often each food is consumed during a given time period. There is evidence in the literature that such questionnaires can validly rank individuals by level of intake of specific nutrients (Newell, et al, 1981). No data exists on the reliability and validity of classifying individuals of different ethnic groups by level of nutrient intake using a single food frequency questionnaire.

FOOD FREQUENCY DEVELOPMENT

Field research has been underway to develop and validate a food frequency questionnaire to ascertain retrospective exposure to dietary factors. The goal of the research is to develop a valid and reliable food frequency questionnaire which characterizes the intake of total fat, vitamin A, and vitamin C intake one year prior to the interview date. Total fat is of interest because of its positive association with the development of breast and colon cancer. Vitamins A and C are inversely associated with lung cancer. Since a food frequency questionnaire must have a food list which includes the population specific food sources of the nutrients of interest, the first step in our research was to inventory the diets of the selected population.

Two south Texas counties were selected which had cancer incidence rates similar to the overall cancer rates in Texas and were representative of the ethnic distribution of Texas. From these counties, 431 men and women, ages 20-60 volunteered to participate in a 24 hour dietary recall interview (Table 2). Data from the 24 hour recall were used to identify the important food sources of the three nutrients. The foods were ranked by their percent

Table 2. Number of Subjects by Ethnic Subgroup and Sex

Sex	Black	Hispanic	White	Total	
Male	21	21	65	107	(25%)
Female	81	77	166	324	(75%)
Total	102 (23%)	98 (23%)	231 (54%)	431	(100%)

contribution to the total intake of each nutrient for each ethnic group (Willet, et al, 1985). Table 3 lists the food types of the total population, ranked by their percent contribution to the total nutrient intake for each nutrient. These food lists were reviewed in order to consolidate all similar food items into single food types. Since a food frequency questionnaire is designed to assess typical or average intake, some specificity in food item descriptions must be forfeited. For instance, all of the types of beef cuts (i.e. steaks, ribs, or roasts) consumed by the population, were grouped into one food type category called beef cuts. Both objective and subjective decisions were made in order to end up with the smallest number of mutually exclusive food types.

Comparison of the ethnic differences in the food list rankings were based on the 25 top ranked, mutually exclusive food types of each ethnic subgroup. The total population list was compared to the list for each ethnic group to determine which food types identified as important nutrient sources for an ethnic group were not enumerated in the total population list. The percent contribution to total fat contributed by the ethnic-specific food types not included in the total population list is shown in Table 4. By using the total population food list, 11.5% of the total

Table 4. The Percent Contribution to Total Fat Intake by the Ethnic-Specific Food Types Not Included in the Total Population List

Black Food Type	%	Hispanic Food Type	%	White Food Type	%
Fried Pork Chop	2.4	Danish Pastry	1.9	Salad Dressing	0.8
Baked or Broiled Chicken	2.3	Taco	1.6		
		Nuts	1.5		
Cakes w/Butter Icing	1.7	Baked or Broiled Chicken	0.7		
Cheese Dishes	1.4				
Bread Stuffing	1.0	Tacito de Cabeza	0.7		
Chicken Stew or Casserole	0.8	Lettuce Salad w/Dressing	0.7		
Rice Cake	0.7				
Fried Fish	0.7				
Cornbread	0.6				
Total	11.5		7.8		0.8

Table 3. Food Types of Total Population Ranked by Percent Contribution

	TOTAL FAT		VITAMIN A		VITAMIN C
	Food Type Name	Percent	Food Type Name	Percent	Food Type Name	Percent
1.	Beef Cuts	9.32	Liver	12.31	Orange Juice	20.01
2.	Ground Beef	3.07	Carrots	10.36	Oranges	7.82
3.	Whole Milk	2.75	Mixed Vegetables	6.22	Kool-Aid, Wylers	6.90
4.	Snack Foods, Chips, Etc.	2.56	Spinach	3.22	Fruitades	2.71
5.	Eggs	2.51	Sweet Potatoes	3.06	Grapefruit	2.31
6.	Sausage	2.10	Greens	2.40	Strawberries	2.13
7.	Butter, Margarine	1.93	Other Cold Cereals	2.38	Lettuce Salad	1.86
8.	Ice Cream	1.70	Eggs	1.85	Broccoli	1.82
9.	Beef Enchilada	1.61	Lettuce Salad	1.73	Potato-Bld-Mshd-Bkd	1.80
10.	Chili Con Carne	1.32	Chicken Stew/Cass.	1.64	Mixed Fruit	1.79
11.	Bacon	1.27	Whole Milk	1.47	Grapefruit Juice	1.47
12.	Pork Cuts	1.12	High Fortified Cereals	1.44	Aloe Vera	1.43
13.	Pizza	1.03	Spaghetti/Meat Balls	1.34	Cranberry Juice	1.37
14.	Chicken Fried Steak	1.01	Beef Stew	1.33	Spanish Rice	1.06
15.	Cheddar Cheese	1.01	Spanish Rice	0.94	Potato Salad	1.03
16.	Potato Salad	1.00	Ice Cream	0.91	Greens	0.99
17.	Ham & Cheese Sand.	0.92	Tamales	0.90	Banana	0.95
18.	Whipping Cream	0.90	Hot Chili Sauce	0.83	French Fries	0.91
19.	Fried Chicken	0.85	Pizza	0.76	Pizza	0.88
20.	Tamales	0.80	Reducing Beverage	0.74	Spaghetti/Meat Balls	0.85
21.	Barbeque Beef Sand.	0.72	Broccoli	0.69	Tomatoes	0.77
22.	Cookie	0.68	Chunky Soup	0.68	Lemonade	0.76
23.	Eggplant	0.63	Butter, Margarine	0.66	Cabbage/Coleslaw	0.69
24.	Avocado	0.58	Tomatoes	0.60	Whole Milk	0.67
25.	Spaghetti/Meat Balls	0.51	Catsup	0.58	Apple	0.65
	Total	41.90	Total	59.04	Total	63.63

fat intake for Blacks and 7.8% of Hispanics would be lost.
If the food sources found as important only in the total

Table 5. The Percent Contribution to Vitamin A Intake by
the Ethnic-Specific Food Types Not Included in the Total
Population List

Black Food Type	%	Hispanic Food Type	%	White Food Type	%
Pie, Sweet Potatoes or Pumpkin	2.5	Green Beens	1.2	Lowfat Milk	1.4
		Potato Salad	0.6		
		Ham Sandwich	0.6	Whipping Cream	0.9
Sausage Sandwich	1.0	Summer Squash	0.6		
Summer Squash	0.9	Taco	0.6	Vegetable Juice Cocktail	0.8
Hamburger Deluxe	0.7	Mixed Fruit	0.6		
Oatmeal	0.6				
Vegetable Juice Cocktail	0.5			Cheddar Cheese	0.7
Bread Stuffing	0.5				
B-B-Q Beef Sand	0.5				
Total	7.1		4.2		3.8

population were used to determine vitamin A intake, among
Blacks 7.1% of vitamin A intake would be lost, and among
Hispanics 4.2% would be lost (Table 5).

Table 6. The Percent Contribution to Vitamin C Intake by
the Ethnic-Specific Food Types Not Included In the Total
Population List

Black Food Type	%	Hispanic Food Type	%	White Food Type	%
Ham Sandwich	1.2	High For- tified Cereals	1.5	Tamales	1.2
Peaches	1.2			High For- tified Cereals	1.0
Hamburger Deluxe	0.9				
Cauliflower	0.7	Hot Green Peppers	1.1		
Sausage Sandwich	0.7			Cantaloupe	0.8
Other Cold Cuts	0.6	Ham Sandwich	1.1	Beef Stew	0.7
		Summer Squash	0.7	Sweet Green Peppers	0.6
		Green Beans	0.6		
		Liver	0.6		
		Cowpeas	0.6		
		Avocado	0.6		
Total	5.2		6.9		4.2

For vitamin C, 5.2% of the Black and 6.9% of the Hispanic intake would be lost by limiting the food frequency list to food sources that were identified in the total population (Table 6).

ETHNIC CONTRIBUTIONS

The percent of nutrient intake captured by the 25 food types based on the total population data and the ethnic-specific data are summarized in Table 7. Using ethnic-specific food types, it was possible to increase the percentage of each nutrient captured among all three ethnic subgroups. The ethnic-specific food lists included food items which provided substantial contributions to nutrient intake. Since the objective was to create one food frequency questionnaire which represented the important food sources of total fat, vitamin A, and vitamin C for the ethnic subgroups, it was necessary to add these important foods identified by the nutrient-specific ranking lists for each of the subgroups with the list for the total population.

Table 7. Improvement in Percent Nutrient Intake by Including Ethnic-Specific Foods

Ethnic Group	TOTAL FAT		VITAMIN A		VITAMIN C	
	Total Population	Ethnic	Total Population	Ethnic	Total Population	Ethnic
White	41.5	42.3	59.4	63.2	56.2	60.4
Black	48.1	59.6	71.6	78.7	74.5	79.7
Hispanic	46.2	54.0	74.4	78.6	71.0	77.9

At this time this food frequency questionnaire is being tested in two new populations in the same two counties to determine its reliability and validity. This food frequency questionnaire will also be evaluated to determine whether the addition of these ethnic-specific food sources changes the classification of individuals quantiled by their intake using just the total population food list.

In summary, the data indicates that ethnic differences do exist in food sources of nutrients that would not be

identified in the list of foods based on the nutrient
intake of the total population. The results show 30 unique
food types from the ethnic-specific lists which were not
identified in the rankings of foods contributing to the
total population for the three nutrients of interest.
Eight of these food types were sources of total fat, 14
were sources of vitamin A, and eight were sources of
vitamin C. In a heterogeneous population, the exclusion of
subgroup specific food sources of nutrients could reduce
the probability of detecting true differences in nutrient
intake of the subgroups, thus biasing the results of the
analysis, by providing inaccurate exposure status data.

REFERENCES

Batcher OM, Nichols JM (1984). Identifying important food
    sources of nutrients. J Nutr Ed 16:177-181
Bazzare TL, Myers MP (1980). The collection of food intake
    data in cancer epidemiology studies. Nutr Cancer
    1(4):22-45
Block G (1982). A review of validations of dietary
    assessment methods. Am J Epid 115:492-505
Committee on Diet, Nutrition, and Cancer (1982). Assembly
    of Life Sciences, National Research Council, National
    Academy of Sciences: Diet, Nutrition and Cancer.
    Washington, DC, National Academy Press
Doll R, Peto R (1981). The causes of cancer. Quantitative
    estimates of avoidable risks of cancer in the United
    States today. J Natl Cancer Inst 66:1191-1308
Macdonald EJ, Heinze EB (1978). Epidemiology of cancer in
    Texas: Incidence analyzed by type, ethnic group, and
    geographic location. New York, Raven Press
Newell GR, Boutwell WB (1981). Cancer differences among
    Texas ethnic groups - An hypothesis. Cancer Bull
    33:113-114
Willet, et al (1985). Reproducibility and validity of a
    semiquantitative food frequency questionnaire. Am J Epid
    122:51-65

Advances in Cancer Control: The War on Cancer—
15 Years of Progress, pages 263–281
© 1987 Alan R. Liss, Inc.

METHODOLOGICAL DEVELOPMENT OF DIETARY FIBER INTERVENTION
TO LOWER COLON CANCER RISK

E E Ho, Jan R. Atwood, Frank L. Meyskens, Jr.

Cancer Prevention and Control Program, Arizona
Cancer Center (EEH and FLM), and College of
Nursing (JRA), University of Arizona, Tucson,
Arizona 85724

INTRODUCTION

Increasing dietary fiber intake to lower colon
cancer risk has been recommended by the National Cancer
Institute (Greenwald 1984), American Cancer Society (ACS
1984) and other organizations committed to cancer
prevention/health promotion. However, several
methodological concerns need to be considered before
dietary fiber intervention can be implemented to achieve
the maximum public health benefit with the least cost and
risk. In this chapter, dietary fiber intervention issues
including risk reduction, cost-effectiveness of
intervention method, and safety will be addressed. Two
algorithms for decision making in the feasibility and
efficacy testing of cancer control interventions will be
presented. The dietary fiber intervention will be used
to illustrate the sequential steps and the implications
of the results.

METHODOLOGICAL ISSUES IN FIBER INTERVENTION

The first methodological concern in dietary fiber
intervention is whether significant risk reduction (e.g.
lowering colon cancer mortality) can be achieved by
increasing certain types of dietary fiber intake in a
population currently consuming a low fiber diet. It is
well documented that various types of fibers and their
fractions exert different physiological and biochemical
effects (Vohouny and Kritchevsky 1981). The protective

role of a specific fiber in colon carcinogenesis can only be established by the results of prospective randomized clinical trials or similarly well controlled experiments, the knowledge of which will not be available for at least several years. Meanwhile, suggestions for types of fiber to eat and how much to eat need to be extrapolated from non-experimental epidemiological observations and experimental animal studies. If methodological studies can demonstrate consumer acceptability of the fiber source at a certain dose level, then the particular fiber intervention may be recommended as one of several viable means of dietary fiber intervention, each with estimated risk reduction.

The second concern is the cost-effectiveness of a chosen intervention method. The same nutritional intervention agent and dose can be delivered by a variety of methods to the subjects. Methodological studies which assess perceptions toward each alternative method, estimate operational costs and determine expected units of impact, will provide crucial information for choosing the most cost-effective and feasible intervention method. It is helpful to recognize that the same dietary intervention method used as a therapeutic regimen may have different effectiveness when used as a disease prevention/health promotion practice. A different set of motivations, beliefs, barriers and benefits may even be involved in the compliance behavior of cancer prevention in comparison to cardiovascular prevention.

Third, whenever a single nutrient or nutritional component is used as a disease prevention agent, cautions should be taken to avoid side effects resulting from overdose or from imbalance of the overall nutritional status. Methodologic studies which monitor the severity and distributuion of potential side effects, identify subject correlates, and test methods of controlling for the side effects are important for further decision making based on the risk/benefit ratio in the target population.

SEQUENTIAL DECISION MAKING

The five phases of cancer control developed by the National Cancer Institute, including hypothesis generation, feasibility testing, efficacy testing, population trial and community demonstration, provide a framework for a progressive approach to cancer control progams (Greenwald and Cullen 1985). The methodological development discussed in this paper will focus on the decision making process involved in the feasibility and efficacy testing of the fiber intervention (Phases II and III). Two algorithms adapted from Lopez's algorithms for nutrition intervention (Lopez, 1986) will be used to illustrate the essential steps in the sequential series of methodological studies (see Figures 1 and 2). A dietary fiber intervention to lower colon cancer risk in a retirement community will be used to illustrate the steps involved in such an approach.

The initiation of a nutritional intervention study (i.e. Cancer Control Phase II Trial) may be decided by following the algorithm in Fig. 1. Evaluation of the scientific evidence of the protective effect of the intervention agent against a particular cancer is only the first step. Review of the relative significance of the specific cancer problem in terms of morbidity and mortality in the target population will assist in prioritizing various cancer sites for cancer control program planning (Namboodiri et al. 1986). Information on the estimated risk reduction with a specific intervention method is important in predicting its public health impact, given a significant cancer problem. Sometimes an intervention with modest reduction in relative risk may be justified if the cancer problem is severe enough at the community level. Assessment of perceived attitudes, knowledge and behaviors associated with the proposed compliance behavior in the target population provides further crucial information on the feasibility of the intervention. It is desirable to list all feasible intervention alternatives and compare the operational cost per unit of impact. The potential side-effects of an intervention method sometimes outweigh the likely benefit except in populations at high risk for the specific cancer. All of the above factors need to be considered in the initiation of a pilot intervention trial.

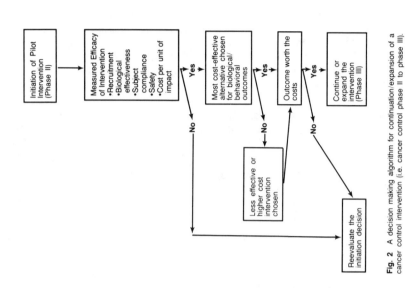

Fig. 2 A decision making algorithm for continuation/expansion of a cancer control intervention (i.e. cancer control phase II to phase III).

Fig. 1 A decision making algorithm for initiation of a nutritional intervention to lower cancer risk (i.e. a cancer control phase II study).

The continuation/expansion of a nutritional intervention (i.e. Cancer Control Phase III Trial) may follow the decision making algorithm in Fig. 2. The efficacy of a specific intervention method needs to be measured in terms of subject recruitment, biological effectiveness in cancer risk reduction, behavioral compliance to the regimen and the dosing schedule, safety from toxic or deleterious effects, and acceptable unit cost for future populations based intervention. Not all pilot studies are designed to measure all aspects of the efficacy issue at the same time. In addition, significant demands on human and physical resources may preclude comprehensive studies from taking place even when the research design provides the framework for it. Often the methodological problems involved in developing reliable and valid measures of one aspect of efficacy (e.g. biological markers of cancer risk) would require extensive resources to carry out. Ideally, pilot data from all aspects of intervention efficacy should be acceptable, and cost-effectiveness and cost/benefit analyses performed before the intervention is continued or expanded into a Cancer Control Phase III trial.

It is not uncommon for community cancer prevention programs to skip the decision making steps outlined in the algorithms. Due to the behavioral/educational focus of some programs, it is understandable that the biological effectiveness of each recommended dietary change in lowering cancer risk is assumed rather than tested. However, the intermediate behavioral outcome needs to be measured, the potential nutritional risk in subpopulations monitored, and cost-benefit analyses conducted. Evaluation of existing programs may also utilize the same algorithms to put current activities into perspective, to identify areas of planning needs, and to expand successful components. Two goals directed our approach to methodology development in dietary fiber intervention. One was to develop a clinical trial model with a single fiber source, so the hypothesis of a causal relationship between the specific fiber and colon cancer risk can be tested. The other goal was to develop the "how-tos" for the general public in following the recommendation to double current fiber intake. A description of the process involved for the fiber intervention will follow below.

INITIATION OF FIBER INTERVENTION

Steps in Fig. 1 are used to illustrate the sequential decision making process in the initiation of a fiber intervention.

Review of Evidence, Significance and Risk Reduction

Based on literature review of the cumulative evidence from epidemiological studies, animal experiments and the proposed mechanisms of action, the National Cancer Institute issued the public recommendation of doubling current dietary fiber intake for Americans to lower colon cancer risk (Greenwald 1984). The significance of colon cancer prevention is self-evident: (1) colon cancer continues to be one of the leading causes of cancer deaths in males and females in the U.S., (2) in the 50% of patients who have advanced colon cancer at the time of diagnosis, the 5-year survival rate is poor (GI Tumor Study Group 1984). Dietary modifications will complement screening for high risk individuals with precancerous lesions. The NCI estimated that 50% reduction in cancer of the colon and rectum could be achieved by the year 2000, with dietary modifications emphasizing fiber-rich foods and reducing fats (Greenwald and Sondik 1986). Whether there is sufficient scientific evidence for the policy recommendation remains a controversial issue among scientists and some consumer groups, and is beyond the scope of this paper. Despite the controversy, an array of cancer education and health promotion organizations has started dietary education program nationally.

The older adult was chosen as the target population for our dietary fiber intervention because of their increased risk of developing precancerous colonic polyps with age. Epidemiological data on migrants suggest that it is possible to change the risk of colon cancer in a lifetime (Correa and Haenszel 1978). From the carcinogenesis perspective, a 15 to 20 year latency period is required and the promotional stage is dose and time dependent. With the life expectancy of Americans increasing into the seventies, and the median age of diagnosis and death from colon cancer in the seventies, intervention starting at early retirement age may have several decades to exert its effect. Therefore, reduction in colon cancer mortality in older adults should be achievable by dietary modifications including fiber intervention.

Evaluation of Alternative Dietary Interventions

Goal oriented literature search focusing on cost benefit/effectiveness ratios of alternative interventions provides the necessary information for this evaluation process.

Fiber vs. Other Dietary Risk Factors. Many dietary components other than fiber have been associated with colon cancer, including fat, B-carotene, Vitamin C, Vitamin E, etc. (NRC 1982). The non-proportional distribution of fiber, fat and micronutrients in foods, and the vast difference in volume of their purified forms, make it necesary to plan for each intervention individually (e.g. a high fiber intake does not follow automatically with a low fat or high vegetable/fruit intake). Feasibility factors such as participant compliance, resource requirements, promptness of behavioral change and generalizability to the public also vary with each dietary intervention. All of these nutritional changes may cumulatively provide a protective effect against cancer.

Fiber Supplementation vs. Changing Total Dietary Fiber. There are various ways of doubling dietary fiber consumption, including increasing intake from various food sources, and supplementation and fortification with a single concentrated source. The chemopreventive approach using a single fiber supplement will require less behavioral change, and is likely to produce better compliance and prompter risk reduction. It is, therefore, an attractive alternative for high risk populations, such as older individuals with history of colonic adenomatous polyps. For the general public it is, of course, desirable to aim at a comprehensive dietary improvement in the long term. In the case of

fiber, the intake of a concentrated source of cereal
fiber can be a first step and an intergral part of a high
fiber diet plan.

Selection of a Fiber Supplement. In the case that
supplementation is the selected method of intervention,
its selection should be based on (1) scientific evidence
of its effectiveness in risk reduction , and (2)
long-term consumer acceptability including taste,
convenience, cost, and daily dose. Any product that
meets the above two criteria may be considered a viable
intervention agent. Among the natural sources of fiber,
wheat bran fiber has been shown to be associated with
reduced colon cancer incidence in rat studies (Reddy and
Wynder 1984) and in epidemiologic studies (McKeown-Eyssen
and Bright-See 1984). The consumer acceptability of the
wheat bran fiber cereal is demonstrated by the
availability of commercial products on the market since
the 1940's. In addition, reports of market surveys
suggest that, as a food category, commercial wheat bran
cereals were used most commonly in older adult households
(Sellery 1984). Once the methodology for wheat bran
fiber supplementation in a target population is
developed, it may be adapted to other sources of fiber
(e.g. rye or oat) shown to be protective for different
targeted populations.

Feasibility Surveys in Target Population

To gain specific information on attitudes,
knowledge, and behavior of a target intervention
population, a randomized survey of a probability sample
of the population is useful in providing baseline data
for program planning. Based upon the knowledge of
attitudes, beliefs and behavior associated with the
proposed intervention in the target population, the
overall participation of the intervention may be
projected.

The feasibility of the chosen dietary intervention
method is assessed by developing valid and reliable test
instruments (Atwood, 1986). Three instruments, Health

Behavior Questionnaire (HBQ), (Atwood et al. 1986), Colon Cancer Prevention Questionnaire (CCPQ), (Ho et al. 1986a) and Dietary Modification for Cancer Prevention Questionnaire (DMCPQ), (Ho et al. 1986b), were developed based on criterion variables in a Health Behavior for Cancer Prevention Model (Atwood et al. 1984), as listed in Table 1. In addition, the format of ethnographic interviews and focus group discussions was developed to further investigate unclear issues or discrepant findings from previous surveys. The instruments and methods described above may be used singularly or in combination as a needs assessment process in community dietary improvement programs.

Table 1: A table of test instruments and their criterion variables (based on Health Behavior in Cancer Prevention Model, Atwood et al. 1985)

Health Behavior Questionnaire (Atwood et al. 1986)
       .efficacy (personal and treatment)
       .health locus of control
       .health threat (severity and susceptibility)
       .health status (general)
       .personal characteristics (age, sex, education)
       .social support
       .value orientation

Colon Cancer Prevention Questionnaire (Ho et al. 1986a)
       .efficacy (personal and treatment)
       .health status (bowel function, food and medication
         use)
       .knowledge about colon ca.
       .social support
       .threat reduction (benefits and barriers)

Dietary Modification for Cancer Prevention Questionnaire (Ho et al. 1986b)
       .health status (food intake patterns)
       .efficacy (personal and treatment)
       .threat reduction (benefits and barriers)
       .social support

Ethnographic Interviews (Benedict et al. 1987)
       .knowledge about dietary modification
       .threat reduction (barriers)

In a mail survey of a retirement community in southern Arizona (Ho et al. 1986a), questionnaires were sent out to a probability sample of the population randomly selected from the phone book. Two survey instruments, the HBQ and the CCPQ, were included in the mail package which was adapted from the personalized method of Dillman (1978). The survey was completed in three months, had a return rate of 48%, and cost about $3,000. Findings directly applicable to the implementation of a fiber intervention trial are summarized below:

Personal Efficacy of the Fiber Intervention. When subjects were presented with a list of alternative methods to increase daily dietary fiber intake, the most favorable choices were overall dietary fiber increase, fiber pills, and fiber cereals. The perceived ability to follow the self selected high fiber plan for a minimun of four years was high (see Table 2). The major reasons given for unwillingness to participate in a fiber intervention were: lack of persuasive scientific evidence, behavioral inconvenience, old age and health barriers.

Table 2: Personal efficacy toward increasing dietary fiber intake by a method of own choice (% of subjects, N=328) (Ho, et al. 1986a)

	yes	no	don't know
could follow	76.2	14.7	9.1
want to participate	43.2	41.2	14.6

Correlates of Personal Efficacy and Implications for Compliance. Knowledge about colon cancer was found to be the best predictor for the subjects' perceived ability and willingness to increase dietary fiber intake to lower colon cancer risk (p 0.001 and p 0.01 for each dependent variable in step-wise multiple regression analysis). Current use of high fiber bran cereals is also a good predictor (p 0.05 for ability and p 0.01 for willingness). The presence of current bowel function problems is associated with the willingness to participate in the intervention (p 0.05), but not the perceived success in such a program. Overall, these findings suggest that educational efforts to increase colon cancer related knowledge may improve participation in and compliance to the fiber intervention.

Perceived Compliance Enhancers and Detractors.
Profiling the relevant compliance enhancers and barriers
of a specific intervention is crucial to ensure maximum
compliance given the resources available. Table 3
summarizes the subjects's perception toward various
compliance related factors observed in the mail survey.

Table 3: Benefits and barriers of increasing dietary fiber
intake by a method of own choice (% of subjects, N-328) (Ho
et al. 1986a)

	positive effect	negative effect	no effect or don't know
convenience	61.3	7.4	31.3
improve bowel movement	55.7	2.5	41.8
effect on health	61.4	1.5	37.0
effect on bowel cancer risk	54.6	0.3	45.1
influence of family/ friends	12.6	2.5	84.9
taste	35.4	3.7	60.9

Compliance Enhancement Activities Perceived Helpful.
In designing a cost-effective compliance enhancement
program for any specific intervention, a survey of the
target population's perceptions of potential activities
can provide information on the general interest and its
distribution. A list of preferred compliance enhancement
activities in the target population was compiled from the
mail survey.

Results of other pilot studies using the DMCPQ and
qualitative methods also contributed to the decision
making process. Pilot testing of the DMCPQ in thirty
older individuals from a residential community (Ho et al.
1986b) suggested that dietary fiber is considered good
for health in general, but its association with colon
cancer risk is not known to many. Different levels of
ability and willingness to follow specific dietary
recommendations were also observed. Use of whole grain
products, fruits and vegetables were viewed as easier and
more likely than lowering fat intake. Approximately one
third of the participants did not know if they were
following a low fat diet in contrast to the three per
cent who did not know about a high fiber diet.

Qualitative methods (Spradley 1979) including ethnographic interviews and focus group discussions were used to further investigate the subjects' perceptions within the contextual perspective (Benedict et al. 1987). Measures were taken to ensure the validity and reliability of the results. Areas of knowledge gap and compliance barriers identified complemented findings of quantitative methods. Together, the above qualitative information suggests that individual dietary changes are more likely to be achieved with adequate knowledge of diet and cancer, reasonable estimation of the difficulties of behavioral change, and attitudes conducive to the modification.

Estimation of Cost, Risk and Benefit

Cost/benefit to society and risk/benefit to the individual are additional items to be considered in the development of a nutritional intervention. However, the decision of whether the likely outcome would be worth the cost and risk is the least objective of all steps involved in the algorithm. All benefit estimates for interventions are necessarily based on insufficient or crude data, and the impact on the quality of life is difficult to quantify. Weinstein (1983) had estimated that the cost of nutritional supplementation in the general public would compare favorably with currently accepted costs of cancer screening. The cost per participant and the cost per incremental improvement in outcome varies a great deal with any recommended dietary behavioral change, depending on the delivery model (e.g. professional counseling, group lessons, self-help groups, peer teaching, and mass media campaign).

The acceptability of side effects for an individual needs to be evaluated in light of the degree of cancer risk reduction expected given the initial at-risk level. The general rule is the higher the initial risk level and the more the estimated risk reduction, the more side effects posed by the agent will be tolerable. In the case of doubling fiber intake with supplements or overall dietary increase, some degree of gastro-intestinal symptoms is not uncommon. A upper limit of dietary fiber intake of 35 grams daily has been suggested by the NCI, considering the potential side effects on mineral balance and metabolism of other nutrients, (Light 1987).

EXPANSION OF THE FIBER INTERVENTION

To obtain efficacy information for decision making of a proposed intervention protocol as outlined in Fig. 2, a pilot study of short duration may be used. A comprehensive compliance enhancement program which addresses major compliance enhancers and barriers may be an integral part of the intervention protocol. Variables perceived to affect subject compliance may also be measured before and after the trial to test the specific impact of individual compliance enhancement strategies.

Measuring the Efficacy of Fiber Supplementation

In our pilot intervention study, an experiment was designed to test the hypothesis that the group with the most comprehensive compliance enhancement program, although having a higher operational cost than less intensive programs, would have the most cost-effectiveness in terms of subject compliance. Subjects who returned previous mail surveys were recruited and randomly assigned to one of the following three treatment groups for three months:

Group A: Fiber Supplement + Education
Group B: Fiber Supplement only
Group C: Control

Group C received the minimal amount of compliance enhancement support in the form of information sharing. Subjects in Groups A and B received further compliance enhancement support in the form of free fiber supplements in an effort to improve treament efficacy. Group A also received a comprehensive educational program developed to meet the needs of general compliance maintenance and individualized problem solving. Results of feasibility surveys in the target population were found to be informative and useful in designing the intervention at this stage. Major findings are summarized below:

Recruitment Methodology. A recruitment technique was developed which used telephone interviews with subjects who returned questionnaires in the previous community mail survey. The interview used a social marketing approach (Novelli 1985) which provided behavioral motivation and emphasized individual contribution. The recruitment of 180 eligible subjects was completed in two months with less than $1,000 expenditure. The combined drop out rate in the three treatment groups was less than 20%. This technique produced an entrant/contact ratio of about 1:4 as compared to ratios between 1:22 to 1:119 in major long-term clinical trials (Tangrea 1984, Hunninghake et al. 1982). The recruitment method validated in this short-term trial may be adapted to be a cost-effective alternative in long-term studies.

Dietary Fiber Intake. Baseline mean daily dietary fiber intake, as estimated by a revised version of the National Cancer Institute's Food Frequency Questionnaire (Block 1986), was similar in the three groups (16.7 +/- 6.9 grams). This consumption level was more than the American mean of 10-15 grams (Murphy and Calloway 1986). The target population could further increase, about 10 grams, daily dietary fiber intake to reach the NCI's goal of 20-35 grams daily. The self-reported mean supplemental dietary fiber intake in subjects staying on the regimen was about 13g in both Groups A and B. At the end of the study, the mean daily dietary fiber intake of these subjects was about 30 grams. In Group C, only four subjects reported increased daily dietary fiber intake of more than two grams. It appeared that a significantly higher level of fiber intake is unlikely to be achieved by dissemination of information alone in the target population.

Compliance Rate and Side Effects. Table 4 lists the compliance rates and side effects of the three treatment groups. "Compliance rate to study participation" refers to the proportion of subjects who completed the study forms before and after the intervention. "Compliance rate to daily regimen intake" designates the proportion of participants who consumed any amount of fiber supplements on a daily basis. In both Groups A and B, subjects who chose to stay on the regimen seemed to self-adjust to a tolerable dose based on convenience and side effects. It appeared that compliance to study participation, to a daily regimen intake and to the recommended dose of that regimen are different parameters of the compliance behavior likely to be influenced by various combinations of factors.

Table 4: Compliance rate, side effects and operational cost of the three treatment groups in the fiber supplementation study (Ho et al. 1986c)

	GROUP A Fiber+ Education (N=60)	GROUP B Fiber only (N= 60)	GROUP C Control (N=60)
.compliance rate to study participation	75%	56%	76%
.compliance rate to daily regimen intake	90%	56%	7%
.rate of intermittent flatulence (regimen compliers only)	60%	93%	80%
.total operational cost	$3,000	$2,000	$360
.operational cost per regimen complier	$51	$66	$91

In Group A subjects who volunteered for blood tests (N=35), there were no observable patterns of change in self-reported body weight, serum cholesterol, triglyceride, high density lipoprotein, CBC, urine analysis and other SMA 20 parameters except for calcium after three months of intervention. The most prevelant gastro-intestinal side effect was intermittent flatulence, diarrhea, and/or constipation. Serum calcium dropped significantly (p 0.01) at the end of the study in one third of subjects tested. Preliminary analysis did not indicate any significant associations of dietary intake of calcium, fiber and protein with the serum calcium change. Until the interaction of minerals and fiber is understood better, it is important to ensure the adequate intake of calcium and other similarly absorbed minerals (e.g. zinc, copper, magnesium) when recommending a high fiber diet. Findings on side effects from this pilot intervention study are critical for designing protocols that minimize side effects in further fiber intervention at the population level.

Cost-effectiveness of the Compliance Enhancement Program. The results supported the hypothesis that a

well-planned compliance enhancement program for the fiber
intervention was most cost-effective for the unit of
impact (i.e. compliant subject). Although the total
operational cost of the control group was the lowest, the
effect on individual behavioral change was also the
smallest. The ready availability of the supplements in
Group B led to a seven fold leap in compliance. An
additional cost of $1,000 (i.e. about an additional $50
per recruited subject) for implementing a comprehensive
compliance enhancement program in Group A resulted in
almost doubling regimen compliance and a modest decrease
in the incidence of gastrointestinal side effects, as
compared to Group B.

   Pilot Testing the Efficacy of Increasing Total
Dietary Fiber Intake. The efficacy of increasing total
dietary fiber intake was tested in 46 older volunteers by
using a teaching module designed for training of peer
counselors. Both low and middle/high socio-economic
status participants demonstrated a significant increase
in knowledge, and indicated the willingness, capability
and intention to carry out the behavioral change.
Comparison of dietary data collected with different
instruments from the same individuals suggested that
repeated 24-hour food records before and after the
intervention would be less subject to participant
reporting bias than food frequency checklists.

IMPLICATIONS

   The decision making strategy in the initiation and
continuation/expansion of a nutritional intervention to
lower cancer risk (Figs. 1 and 2) was demonstrated to be
practical in our sequential approach of dietary fiber
intervention for colon cancer prevention. It is
applicable to general cancer control strategy and
community health promotion programs. Techniques used in
this process, including goal oriented literature search
focusing on cost/benefit ratios of alternative
interventions, development of valid and reliable
instruments to assess health behavior related to
intervention methods in the target population, survey of
the feasibility of the proposed intervention and
potential enhancers and detractors to compliance, and
pilot studies to assess different aspects of the efficacy

of the intervention also have general implications for cancer control programs.

Results from the feasibility studies and the intervention study have been used by the Cancer Prevention and Control Program at the Arizona Cancer Center to (1) develop the clinical protocol for a Phase II cancer control chemoprevention trial (i.e. using wheat bran fiber supplementation in patients with adenomatous colonic polyps and (2) develop a cost-effective delivery model of community-wide nutritional intervention for cancer prevention/health promotion.

REFERENCES

American Cancer Society (1984). Nutrition and cancer: causes and prevention. ACS Special Report, CA: A Cancer Journal for Clinicians 34:121-126.

Atwood JR, Hurd PD, Sheehan ET, Ho E, Sievers JA (1985). Theoretical model development: health behavior in cancer prevention. Nursing Research, 34(6):385. (abstract).

Atwood JR, Hurd PD, Sheehan ET, Ho E, Sievers JA (1986). Health behavior in cancer prevention: model and instruments. Presented at 114th Annual Meeting, American Public Health Association, Las Vegas, (abstract).

Benedict J, Atwood JR, Ho E (1987). An inductive investigation of the elderly's perceptions of diet and cancer prevention. Am Public Health Association, New Orleans.

Block G, Hartman AM, Dresser C, Carroll MD, Gannon J, Gardner L (1986). A data-based approach to diet questionnaire design and testing. Am J of Epidemiology 124(3):453-469.

Correa P, Haenszel W (1978). The epidemiology of large-bowel cancer. In Klein G, Weinhouse S (eds): "Advances in Cancer Research," Vol. 26.

Dillman DA (1978). "Mail and Telephone Survey: The Total Design Method". John Wiley & Sons, Inc.

Doll R, Peto R (1981). "The Causes of Cancer". New York: Oxford University Press.

Greenwald P. Sondik EJ, eds (1986). Cancer control objectives for the nation 1985 - 2000. (in press). US Dept of Health and Human Services, Public Health Service, NIH, NCI, Bethesda.

Greenwald P (1984). Dietary fiber and lowering colon cancer risk. A Statement from the Director's Office, Division of Cancer Prevention and Control. National Cancer Institute.

Greenwald P, Cullen J (1985). The new emphasis in cancer control. JNCI 74(3).

Ho E, Abrams C, Atwood J, Meyskens FL (1986). Health attitudes and behaviors of the elderly toward dietary modification for colon cancer prevention. Presented at Annual Meeting of the American Society of Clinical Oncology, Los Angeles, (abstract).

Ho E, Sievers JA, Abrams C, Meyskens FL (1986). A questionnaire to assess health attitudes, beliefs and behavior related to interim dietary guidelines for reducing cancer risk. Presented at American Society of Preventive Oncology, (abstract).

Ho E, Abrams C, Meyskens FL (1986). Wheat bran fiber supplementation for colon cancer prevention: a feasibility study in the elderly. Presented at 14th International Cancer Congress, Budapest, Hungary, (abstract).

Hunninghake D, Peterson F, LaDouceur M, Knoke J, Leon A (1982). Recruitment from clinical studies. Circulation 66(suppl IV):IV:15-19.

Lanza E (1987). Diet and cancer. In "The Surgeon General's Report on Diet and Health", US Dept of Health and Human Services. (in press).

Light L (1987). Healthy eating to lower cancer risk. (in press). Promoting Health, Am Hosp Assoc. Chicago.

Lopez LM (1986). Evaluating the evidence for nutrition interventions: two algorithms. J of the Am Dietetic Association 86(8):1055-1058.

McKeown-Eyssen GE, Bright-See E (1984). Dietary factors in colon cancer: international relationships. Nutrition and Cancer 6(3):160-70.

Murphy SP, Calloway DH (1986). Nutrient intakes of women in NHANES II, emphasizing trace minerals, fiber and phytate. Research 86(10):1366-1372.

Namboodiri KK, Cavalaris CJ, Tewart BE (1986). A framework for cancer control planning and priority setting. paper presented at International Cancer Congress. Budapest, Hungary.

National Academy of Sciences (1982). "Diet, Nutrition and Cancer Prevention." National Academy Press.

Novelli WD (1985). Social marketing and dietary cancer
prevention. In Greenwald P, Ershow AG, Novelli WD
(eds): "Cancer, Diet and Nutrition: A comprehensive
Sourcebook," Chicago: Marquis Who's Who, Inc.

Patterson WB (1983). Oncology perspective on colorectal
cancer in the geriatric patient. In Yancik R (ed):
"Perspectives on Prevention and Treatment of Cancer in
the Elderly," New York: Raven Press.

Reddy BS, Wynder EL (1984). Primary prevention of colon
cancer: an interdisciplinary approach. CA: A Cancer
Journal for Clinicians.

Sellery SB (1984). New product opportunities: diet for
older Americans. J of Nutrition for Elderly
4(1):31-41.

Spradley JP (1979). "The Ethnographic Interview." New
York: Holt, Rinehart and Winston.

Tangrea J (1984). Recruitment: a perspective for
multicenter clinical trials. Chemoprevention clinical
trials; problems and solutions, NIH Publication No.
85-2715:30-32.

Vahouny GV, Kritchevsky D (eds) (1981). "Dietary Fiber
in Health and Disease." New York:Plenum Press.

Weinstein M (1983). Cost-effective priorities for cancer
prevention. Science 2:17-23.

Wynder EL, Gori GB (1977). Contribution of the
environment to cancer incidence: an epidemiologic
exercise. JNCI 58:825-32.

This paper was supported by the Cancer Center Core Grant
of the Arizona Cancer Center #CA 23074, the Arizona Disease
Commission Block Grant #8277-000000-1-1-ZH-7498, the Robert
S. Flinn Medical Research Grant and the University of
Arizona Basic Research Support Grant.

Advances in Cancer Control: The War on Cancer—
15 Years of Progress, pages 283–287
© 1987 Alan R. Liss, Inc.

MITOXANTRONE SALVAGE IN HEAVILY PRETREATED ADVANCED BREAST
CANCER

L. Nathanson and M.E. Williams

Winthrop-University Hospital and Nassau
Regional CCOP, Mineola, NY   11501 and SUNY
at Stony Brook, Stony Brook, NY   11790

INTRODUCTION

An extensive literature now exists on the use of the
aminoanthaquinone mitoxantrone in human malignancy
(Nathanson, 1984). Studies of the drug as a single agent
in breast cancer have produced variable results. In a
study carried out by the Southwest Oncology Group, 6 objective responses were seen in a total of 92 patients (7%),
but among those patients who were in a "good risk" category,
there were 3 responses in 23 patients (14%) (Stephens,
1983). When mitoxantrone was used as a first line agent in
advanced breast cancer, an objective response rate of 15%
was achieved (Wilson, 1984). In an interesting study of
patient acceptability, where mitoxantrone and doxorubicin
were compared, the great majority of patients preferred the
former drug because of milder GI toxicity. (Stuart-Harris,
1986). Review of the literature demonstrates that although
mitoxantrone has significant cardiotoxicity, it is less
toxic than doxorubicin. Most episodes of cardiotoxicity
reported occurred in prior recipients of doxorubicin
(Nathanson , 1984). The current study attempted to assess
the efficacy and toxicity of mitoxantrone used as a single
agent in metastatic breast cancer patients who were heavily
pretreated and had drug resistant tumor.

MATERIALS AND METHODS

Nine patients with advanced breast cancer were treated.
Median age was 67 (range 48 - 81). Performance status-
mean 1-2 (range 0 - 3). Prior number of chemotherapy

regimens was 2 (range 2 - 6). All patients had previously
received doxorubicin. Prior total doxorubicin dose was
median 290 mg (range 95 - 680mg) with a dose per m^2 BSA of
193 (range 58 - 378). Pretreatment ejection fractions
ranged from 52% to 82%, all of which were considered within normal limits. Sites of measureable metastases in these
patients included soft tissue (3), bone (6), liver (1),
lung or pleura (2). Treatment was carried out at 12 mg/m^2
IV q 3 weeks starting dose.

RESULTS

Mean number of treatments was 6.5 (range 1 - 9);
median individual dose delivered was 17.5 mg (range 5 - 25).
Median total dose of mitoxantrone delivered in these
patients was 85 mg (range 30 - 160 mg) or 60 mg/m^2 (range
40 - 102 mg/m^2).

Median time on study to death in 5 patients who have
died was 37 weeks (range 4 - 45 weeks). Median time on
study for 4 patients who are alive was 21+ weeks. Among
the living patients, 2 remain on study, 2 were removed from
study, one because of progression and one because of marrow
aplasia.

A summary of drug toxicity is shown in Table 1.

TABLE 1

TOXICITY **

Decrease in Ejection Fraction		Nadir WBC $(x10^3)$		Nadir Platelet $(x10^3)$		N	V	Alopecia		Stomatitis	
None	2	WNL	1	WNL	5	0	1	0	5	0	6
>20%	1	<4	2	100	1	1	5	1	3	1	2
>40%		<3	1	75	2	2	2	2	1	2	
>60%		<2	5	50		3	1	3		3	
>80%	1*	<1		25		4		4		4	
No Repeat	3										
Too Early	2										

*Congestive Heart Failure May Have Contributed to Patient's Death

**Left Column – Severity of Toxicity⎫
  Right Column – Number of Patients⎬ in each toxic category

In general, toxicity was tolerable and mild, but 1 patient (prior doxorubicin dose 378 mg/m^2) experienced severe diminution of LV ejection fraction, went into congestive failure and died approximately 8 weeks later. Cardiotoxicity probably contributed to her death. Total mitoxantrone dose was 1101.4 mg/m^2 in this patient.

Objective antitumor response is summarized in Table 2.

TABLE 2

OBJECTIVE RESPONSE

	Total	Alive	Duration of Response (months)
CR	0	0	
PR	5	2	5,5,7,7,8
NC	2	1	
Prog	1	0	
Too Early	1	1	

Five of 8 evaluable patients (62%) achieved a partial objective response with median duration of 7 months (range 5 - 8 months). Sites of response included soft tissue lesions in the chest wall (2), bone scan (2), liver scan (1), and disappearance of pleural effusion (1).

DISCUSSION

Somewhat higher mitoxantrone response rates have been reported from Europe. Smith (1983) observed a 36% response rate in non-pretreated, and 22% response rate in pretreated breast cancer patients. Neidhart reported a 35% partial response rate in 52 women, 50 of whom had been heavily pretreated (1983). Mouridsen similarly found responses in 11 of 25 patients (44%) when mitoxantrone was used as a first-line agent (1983). Thus, our study was not significantly different from that of other investigators who have observed considerable antitumor activity in metastatic breast cancer even when those patients appeared to be re-sistant to other chemotherapeutic agents including doxorubicin. It should be noted that our responding patients, especially those with bone disease, experienced gratifying improvement in the quality of their lives.

CONCLUSION

In Heavily Pretreated Advanced Breast Cancer:

1. Single agent mitoxantrone chemotherapy at a dose of 12 mg/m^2 IV q 13 weeks yielded subjective and partial objective responses in 5 of 8 evaluable patients. Sites of response included bone, soft tissue, pleura and possibly liver.

2. Toxicity, including bone marrow suppression (9 of 9), nausea and vomiting (8 of 9), alopecia (4 of 9), and stomatitis and diarrhea (2 of 9), was mild and well tolerated.

3. However, severe cardiotoxicity occurred in 1 patient (total dose mitoxantrone 101.4 mg/m^2) which probably contributed to her death.

REFERENCES

Mouridsen HT, van Oosterom AT, Rose C, Nooi MA (1983). A phase II study of mitoxantrone as first line cytotoxic therapy in advanced breast cancer. Proc 13th Int Cong of Chemotherapy, Vienna, Part 212, 30-34.

Nathanson L (1984). Mitoxantrone. Can Treatment Review 11:289-293.

Neidhart JA, Gochnour D, Roach RW, Young DC (1983). Mitoxantrone versus doxorubicin in advanced breast cancer: A randomized crossover trial. Proc of 13th Int Cong of Chemotherapy, Vienna, Part 212, 26-29.

Smith IE, Stuart-Harris R, and Pavlidis N (1983). Mitoxantrone alone and in combination in the treatment of advanced breast cancer. Proc 13th Int Cong of Chemotherapy, Vienna, Part 212, 23-25.

Stephens, RL, VonHoff DD, Taylor SA, Knight WA, Livingston RB, Bull FE, Cowan J. Hilgers R, Osborne CK, Gates GA, Clark G (1983). Southwest Oncology Group phase II studies with mitoxantrone in nonhematologic malignancies. IN Rozencweig M, VonHoff DD, Staquet MJ (eds) "New Anti-cancer Drugs: Mitoxantrone and Bisantrene". New York: Raven Press pp 125-130.

Stuart-Harris R, Coates AS, Raghaven D, Sullivan A, Kefford R, Tattersall MHN (1986). Patient acceptability of chemotherapy in advanced breast cancer: A randomized crossover study of mitoxantrone versus doxorubicin. Proc AACR, 27:177.

Wilson KS, Paterson AHG (1984). Single agent mitoxantrone as first-line chemotherapy in advanced breast cancer. Proc ASCO 3:117.

Advances in Cancer Control: The War on Cancer—
15 Years of Progress, pages 289–297
© 1987 Alan R. Liss, Inc.

CLINICAL RELEVANCE OF THE CA-125 ASSAY FOR THE MANAGEMENT OF PATIENTS WITH OVARIAN CARCINOMA

R.N. Raju, M.H. Dalbow, R.P. Pugh, J.P.
Concannon, B.L. Zidar, C.F. Zamerilla and L.L.
Schenken
Division Medical Oncology, Allegheny General
Hospital and Allegheny Singer Research Institute,
Pittsburgh, PA 15212

INTRODUCTION

The CA-125 was first recognized by Bast et al (1981) as a tumor associated antigen in ovarian carcinomas. A radioimmunometric assay utilizing monoclonal antibody reagents was developed by Klug et al (1984) for the quantitative measurement of the tumor marker in serum. Circulating levels of CA-125 were measured in serum or plasma specimens of 73 patients with pathologically confirmed ovarian carcinoma. The data obtained were evaluated for diagnostic efficacy in the detection of primary, recurrent and/or metastatic disease. The data indicate the CA-125 is of little value as an indicator of ovarian malignancy in patients with early localized disease. Significant levels of circulating CA-125 were observed in preoperative specimens of patients with advanced lesions.

Several specimens, monitoring disease status, were assayed in 36 patients. Fifteen of the patients had biopsy confirmed recurrent and/or metastatic disease during the monitoring period. Significant elevations and/or rising trends were observed in all patients as little as one month, but as much as nine months, prior to detection by other procedures. Trending of the CA-125 tracks correlated well with a positive or negative clinical response to newly initiated therapy.

The results of this study indicate that the assay for CA-125 may be a valuable addition to the armamentarium of tumor markers available for the management of patients with ovarian carcinoma.

METHODS

Assay Procedure

Commercially available reagent kits (Abbott Laboratories, - N. Chicago, IL 60064) were used for the assay of
CA-125. Complete instructions for the assay procedure are
included in the package insert with each kit. In brief, a
monoclonal antibody highly specific for one reactive site
(antigenic-epitope) on the tumor marker molecule is
immobilized on a bead. The patient's serum or plasma is
added to the bead and the tumor marker is immunologically
bound by the specific antibody. After incubation and wash
a second monoclonal antibody recognizing a different
epitope is added. The second antibody was radio-labeled
with ^{125}I. The quantity of second antibody bound is
dependent on the quantity of tumor marker present in the
patient's serum and the radio-label increases proportionately to the concentration of the tumor marker. A series
of standards containing pre-determined concentrations of
CA-125 are provided with the kits. These standards must be
assayed each time the procedure is run. A standard curve
may be constructed and the concentration of the tumor
marker may be manually determined from the curve. Alterna-
tively computer programmed instruments such as the
Abbott-ANSR will construct the standard curves internally,
integrate the counts of the unknown and print out the tumor
marker concentration.

Populations Examined

The retrospective specimens examined in this study
were obtained from patients randomly selected from patients
who had an initial diagnosis of primary ovarian carcinoma.
The specimens were stored at -20°C in the cancer research
serum bank of the Allegheny Singer Research Institute.
Prospective specimens were assayed as they became
available.

Specimens obtained from asymptomatic individuals (70),
patients with benign diseases (82) and patients with malignancies other than ovarian carcinoma (156) were assayed for
CA-125 so as to establish circulating levels that would be
discriminatory in the diagnosis of patients with ovarian

cancer.

RESULTS

Diagnosis

The CA-125 levels determined for three control groups are shown in Table 1.

TABLE 1. CA-125 LEVELS DETERMINED FOR CONTROL GROUPS.

CATEGORY	No. Studies	CA-125 (units/ml) >35	>65
ASYMPTOMATIC	70	2	1
BENIGN DISEASES	82	30 (36%)	22 (27%)
OTHER MALIGNANCIES	156	47 (30%)	31 (20%)

Substantial elevations in circulating CA-125 were observed in specimens of patients with benign and malignant diseases other than ovarian carcinoma. Males and females were included in these control groups. The number of elevations were not dependent on sex as the distributions were proportionately nearly equal (females - 33%, males -31%). Only female specimens were examined in the asymptomatic control group.

The results of the CA-125 assay levels in specimens obtained from patients with ovarian carcinoma are shown in Table 2 by stage of disease.

TABLE 2. PRETREATMENT CA-125 LEVELS IN PATIENTS WITH OVARIAN CARCINOMA

STAGE	No. Patients	CA-125 (units/ml) >35	>65
I	14	2 (14%)	1 (7%)
II	13	4 (31%)	4 (31%)
III	18	15 (83%)	11 (61%)
IV	28*	25 (89%)	23 (82%)
TOTALS	73	46 (63%)	39 (53%)

*Includes patients with previously treated but newly diagnosed metastic disease.

Significant elevations were rarely observed in the sera of patients with limited localized disease. The data indicate a makedly stage dependent correlation with increasing CA-125 values; suggesting that circulating levels are somewhat related to tumor burden.

Prognosis

The prognostic significance of the preoperative CA-125 serum level was examined in a group of patients who have been followed three or more years. A summary of this analysis may be seen in Table 3.

TABLE 3. PROGNOSTIC SIGNIFICANCE PRE-OP CA-125 LEVEL WITH OVARIAN CARCINOMA.

STAGE	STATUS	PRE-OP CA-125 Units/ml	
		>35	>65
I	CFD	1/7	0/7
	NFD	1/3	1/3
II	CFD	0/5	---
	NFD	4/4	4/4
III	CFD	5/7 (71%)	3/7 (43%)
	NFD	8/9 (88%)	7/9 (78%)

CFD - Clinically Free of Disease
NFD - Not Free of Disease

Monitoring

CA-125 levels were determined in serial specimens of 36 patients with various primary stages of ovarian carcinoma. The serial data were evaluated to determine the degree to which the CA-125 would identify patients with progressive disease and discriminate these patients from patients who remained clinically free of disease. Table 4 shows the details of this analysis.

TABLE 4.   CA-125 MONITORING TREATMENT RESPONSE IN PATIENTS
WITH OVARIAN CARCINOMA

DISEASE STATUS	CA-125 TREND		
	Fluctuating (<35)	Fluctuating (>35)	Rising
CFD	5/21 (24%)*	3/21 (14%)	0/21
Recurrence	--	--	15/15
Progression	--	--	13/13

CFD - Clinically Free of Disease
* - 2 Patients Initial Stage IV

Twenty one of the 36 patients serially monitored for
serum CA-125 levels had no evidence of malignant disease at
the time of this analysis. Fluctuations in the circulating
CA-125 were apparent and three of the paients showed significant transient elevations. Persistant rising trends
however were not observed in the CFD patient group. Treatment failure was signalled in 15 of 15 patients by a
significant rise in the circulating CA-125. A persistent
rising trend was observed in 10 patients over periods as
much as nine months prior to detection of recurrence by
other procedures. Two of the 15 patients in relapse
responded to newly initiated therapy and 13 progressed.
The CA-125 demonstrated a declining trend in the responding
patients while persistent elevations and/or rising trends
were evident in all patients with progressive disease.

DISCUSSION

The criteria for the evaluation of the clinical significance of a tumor marker as listed by Herberman (1982)
have been examined for the relevance of CA-125 in the
management of patients with ovarian carcinoma. The data
indicate that the CA-125 will not fullfil the criteria of
an acceptable diagnostic test. Concannon et al (1973) in
evaluating the CEA assay for the diagnosis of malignant
disease stated that the problem in differential diagnosis
does not reside in discriminating between asymptomatic
individuals and patients with cancer but in distinguishing
patients with benign diseases that mimic cancer from the
patient with cancer. The incidence of 27% CA-125 false
positives in the benign disease group (> 65 U/ml) may be
acceptable if a great proportion of the early malignancies
could be detected at or above this level. The CA-125 fails

to circulate at significant levels in the majority of patients with Figo Stages I and II disease. It is also apparent that the CA-125 although recovered from ovarian tumors (Bast et al - 1981) is not specific for ovarian carcinoma as confirmed in Table 1. The CA-125 may circulate at high levels in patients with primary malignancies of other anatomical sites. This is especially apparent in patients with adenocarcinoma and anaplastic large cell carcinomas of the lung.

Significant CA-125 antigenemia has been observed in patients with mammary carcinoma (Schenken et al 1985) as well as in extracts of breast tumor tissue (Schenken et al 1986).

The limited data shown in Table 3 suggest that the CA-125 may afford the physician with some prognostic information of clinical value perhaps even in deciding upon a more aggressive approach to therapy in those patients with high pre-operative CA-125 levels. Certainly a much broader study is indicated before reaching this conclusion and the CA-125 as well as other clinical data must be considered in correlation with other prognostic factors as discussed by Richardson et al (1985).

There is general concensus that the major clinical value to be gleaned from serum tumor markers is through serial monitoring of patients who have or have had a malignant disease. In this limited study population the CA-125 shows favorably. The sensitivity of assay for detecting relapse was 100% and in the poorest light considering the fluctuating trends the specificity would approximate 86%. One patient who remains CFD has shown major elevations in excess of 100 U/ml on two occasions. This patient has now been followed for more than one year following her last elevation and all metastic workups short of laporatomy have proven negative. The patient is asymptomatic and the CA-125 although elevated has decreased to approximately 40 U/ml. A similar corre- lation of 94% between CA-125 levels and disease status of patients serially monitored following diagnosis of ovarian carcinoma was observed by Bast et al (1984).

There is little debate with the treatise that a reliable serum test would be invaluable provided it impacted on the management of patients with ovarian carcinoma. At present such information may be of little clinical value to the patient or to the physician. Concannon et al (1974) in reviewing the issue of the clinical relevance of CEA monitoring in patients with bronchogenic carcinoma directed attention to the fact that there is little that can be done therapeutically for patients should the CEA signal progressive disease. A similar dilemma exists in the management of patients with ovarian carcinoma. Once a patient has failed induction chemotherapy the salvage rate with second line chemotherapy has been abysmal (Ozols and Young 1984). The Princess Margaret Hospital experience, reported by Dembo et al 1979 and updated by Dembo (1982 and 1984), demonstrating the efficacy of postoperative total abdominal radiotherapy (TAR) in sequential multimodality therapy has fostered a number of trials to evaluate the TAR for chemotherapy failures. These trials as reported by Malcolm et al (1983) and Peters et al (1986) have failed to improve the salvage rate except in a few cases of patients with limited residuum. There is also a high degree of morbidity associated with TAR following intensive chemotherapy.

Ozols et al (1984) have experienced a favorable response in 35% of a series of patients treated by high dose cisplatin following failure on the standard dose. There have been numerous attempts to reduce high dose chemo toxicity which may prove beneficial, but to date there has been little advantage to patients with poor prognostic histology and/or large residual tumor burden. It may be reasonable to conclude that serial monitoring of CA-125 will not benefit the majority of these patients.

The salvage rate would most certainly be higher if the recurrence were amenable to resection. A classic case has been observed in this study. A presurgical CA-125 > 100 U/ml dropped dramatically at 3 months and persisted low for 12 months followed by a steadily rising trend. Second look laptortomy at this time was negative for malignant disease. CT scans at 18 months failed to reveal recurrent or residual disease. The patient presented with abdominal pain at approximately 21 months at which time the CA-125 was measured at 82 U/ml. A third surgical procedure revealed a small mesenteric nodule approximate to the sigmoid which was resected and the patient's CA-125 has normalized since this procedure. This may be the exceptional case but these data are encouraging and suggest the need for including

CA-125 monitoring in all current or newly activated
clinical trials for the treatment of ovarian carcinoma.

In such a prospective study it would be imperative to
compare the predictive value of the CA-125 versus
second-look laporatomy. Richardson et al (1985) have
called attention to the fact that in the best series
(Stuart et al 1982) nearly 30% of the patients declared
free of disease later relapsed. In another series reported
by Ehrmann et al (1980) the laporatomy correctly identified
only 46% of the patients thought to be disease free. It is
possible that the CA-125 may be beneficial in monitoring
patients clinically free of disease and may indicate the
need for the second look procedure only in patients with
rising marker levels. The sensitivity and specificity for
detecting or excluding relapse in this population, however,
must be established.

Acknowledgements: This work was supported in part by a
grant in aide from the Allegheny Singer Research Institute,
Pittsburgh, PA 15212.

REFERENCES

Bast RC, Fenney M, Lazarus H, et al (1981). Reactivity of
    a monoclonal antibody with human ovarian carcinoma. J
    Clin Invest 68:1331-1337.
Bast RC, Klug TL, Schaetal E, et al (1984). Monitoring
    human ovarian carcinoma with a combination of CA-125, CA
    la-a and carcinoembryonic antigen. Am J Obstet Gynecol
    149:553-559.
Concannon JP, Dalbow MH and Frich JC (1973). Carcino-
    embryonic antigen (CEA) plasma levels in untreated
    cancer patients and patients with metastatic disease.
    Radiology 108:191-193.
Concannon JP, Dalbow MH, Liebler GA, et al (1974). The
    carcinoembryonic antigen assay in bronchogenic carci-
    noma. Cancer 34:184-192.
Dembo AJ, Van Dyk J, Japp B, et al (1979). Ovarian carci-
    noma: Improved survival following abdominopelvic
    irradiation in patients with a completed pelvic
    operation. Am J Obstet Gynecol 134:793-800.
Dembo AJ, Bush RS (1982). Choice of postoperative therapy
    based on prognostic factors. Int J Radiat Oncol Biol
    Phys 8:893-897.

Dembo AJ (1984). Radiotherapeutic management of o arian carcinoma. Seminars Oncol 11:238-250.

Ehrman RL, Federschneider JM, Knapp RC (1980). Distinguishing lymph node metastases from benign glandular inclusions in low-grade ovarian carcinoma. Am J Obstet Gynecol 136:737-746.

Herberman RB (1982). "Biochemical Markers in Cancer" New York: Marcel DEKKER, pp. 1-23.

Klug TL, Bast RC, Niloff JM, et al (1984). A monoclonal antibody immunoradiometric assay for an antigenic determinant (CA-125) associated with human epithelial ovarian carcinomas. Cancer Res 44:1048-1053.

Malcolm AW, Hainsworth JD, Johnson DH, et al (1983). Advanced minimal residual ovarian carcinoma: Abdominal pelvic irradiation following combination chemotherapy. Proc Am Soc Clin Oncol 2:151.

Ozols RF, Young RC (1984). Chemotherapy of ovarian cancer. Seminars Oncol 11:251-263.

Ozols RF, Corden BJ, Jacob J, et al (1984). High dose cisplatin in hypertonic saline. Ann Intern Med 100:19-24.

Peters WA, Blasko JC, Bagley CM, et al (1986). Salvage therapy with whole-abdominal irradiation in patients with advanced carcinoma of the ovary previously treated by combination chemotherapy. Cancer 58:880-882.

Richardson GS, Scully RE, Najamosama N, Nelson JH (1985). Common epithelial cancer of the ovary. N Engl J Med 312:415-424.

Schenken LL, Pugh RP, Dalbow MH and Tippett BK (1985). Intercomparison of CEA, CA-125 and CA 19-9 antigen levels in patients with carcinoma of the breast. (Abstract), San Antonio Breast Cancer Symposium, November 1985.

Schenken LL, Pugh RP, Dalbow MH, Tippett BK and Zammerilla CF (1986). Diversity of antigenic expression in patients with breast tumors; serum and tissue levels of CA 19-9, CA-125 and CEA antigens. (Abstract) American Association of Cancer Research Annual Meeting.

Stuart GCE, Jeffries M, Stuart JL, Anderson RJ (1982). The changing role of "second-look" laporatomy in the management of epithelial carcinoma of the ovary. Am J Obstet Gynecol 142:612-616.

Advances in Cancer Control: The War on Cancer—
15 Years of Progress, pages 299–302
© 1987 Alan R. Liss, Inc.

ANTIEMETIC EFFECTS OF METOCLOPRAMIDE (M) CONTINUOUS
INFUSION (CI): SAFETY, EFFICACY, PATIENT PREFERENCE, AND
COST REDUCTION.

C.A. Presant, C. Wiseman, K. Gala, P. Kennedy,
A. Bouzaglou, D. Blayney, J. Schindler, M.
Rigas, J. Melville, J. Dolan, and L. Jund.
Wilshire Oncology Medical Group & Los Angeles
Oncologic Institute, Los Angeles; and Queen of
the Valley Hospital and Oncology Program, West
Covina, California.

INTRODUCTION

Many chemotherapy programs with high degrees of
effectiveness in palliation and high cure rates are
associated with severe nausea and vomiting. Often the
severity of vomiting causes patients to have a marked
decrease in quality of life, and in some cases, even refuse
further treatment. These chemotherapy regimens usually
contain cisplatinum, high doses of cyclophosphamide, or
DTIC. The conventional approaches to controlling nausea
and vomiting usually contain metoclopramide administered by
a bolus injection over 15 to 30 minutes which is repeated
every 2 hours. In many instances, dexamethasone is given
either with metoclopramide or in place of metoclopramide,
and frequently patients receive sedation with diazepam,
lorazepam, or barbiturates.

Metoclopramide has previously been investigated in
pharmacologic trials by continuous intravenous infusion.
(Taylor, 1984) We studied this technique for
metoclopramide administration in order to determine safety
and efficacy of metoclopramide administered as a loading
dose followed by continuous infusion, and to determine
whether patients preferred metoclopramide administered by
continuous intravenous infusion or by bolus administration.
In addition, we surveyed two hospitals to determine the
cost to patients of metoclopramide infusions compared to
metoclopramide conventional bolus administration.

METHODS

In our trial, metoclopramide infusions were initiated by administration of a loading dose of metoclopramide between 1.5 and 4.0 milligrams per kilogram over 15 minutes. This was administered 30 minutes prior to chemotherapy. Following the loading dose, metoclopramide infusions were continued at a dose of 0.3 to 0.68 milligrams per kilogram per hour for a duration of between 4 and 72 hours.

In addition, all patients received hydration with saline diuresis and with mannitol and furosemide for cisplatinum therapy. Also, the patients received chlorpromazine, pentobarbital, and dexamethasone 30 minutes prior to the chemotherapy.

RESULTS

Fourteen patients received 24 infusions of metoclopramide. Six of these 14 patients received metoclopramide only by continuous infusion. However, comparative analyses were possible in 8 patients who received metoclopramide by conventional bolus administration during some courses of chemotherapy, and metoclopramide by the continuous infusion.

Twelve patients received this in an in-patient setting, and 2 patients were treated satisfactorily in an office setting. The chemotherapy in all patients except one involved cisplatinum. In the other patient, high dose cyclophosphamide was being administered in a method which had previously produced severe nausea and vomiting.

Side effects were relatively rare in these patients. All patients had at least mild sedation. Those patients with mild sedation were able to be easily aroused, and at the conclusion of the metoclopramide they were able to awaken easily and proceed with activities of daily living. In three patients there was moderate sedation which resulted in some slight grogginess during the course of the infusion, but following the completion of the infusion they were able to proceed with normal activities. In two patients severe sedation was produced with some degree of grogginess that persisted after the conclusion of the infusion, with some unsteadiness of gait at that time. Two patients had diarrhea that was easily controlled with lomotil, and only one patient had an extrapyramidal reaction occurring 26 hours after initiation of metoclopramide.

In the 14 patients, 11 (79%) had complete control of nausea and vomiting, 3 other patients (21%) had mild vomiting which occurred a maximum of three times during the post chemotherapy period. In the 24 courses of therapy, 18 (75%) were associated with no vomiting but 6 (25%) were associated with some vomiting.

Three patients had anticipatory vomiting prior to initiation of metoclopramide continuous infusion. In 2 of those, the vomiting instantly stopped. In the other patient, the vomiting was instantly improved, although some vomiting persisted for 24 hours after initiation of the infusion. In that patient, the infusion was continued for 48 hours and no vomiting occurred during the final 24 hours of the infusion.

We compared the efficacy of metoclopramide continuous infusions of less than 10 hours duration with those of greater than 10 hours duration. In 9 courses less than 10 hours in duration, 4 (44%) were associated with vomiting. In 15 courses longer than 10 hours, only 2 (13%) were associated with vomiting.

In 8 patients, metoclopramide continuous infusion was the preferred form of metoclopramide administration in 7 patients. In only one patient was the intermittent bolus administration preferred, and that patient preferred bolus administration because she felt that there was less drowsiness associated with the treatment. Of the 7 patients who preferred infusion, 5 had received bolus injection of metoclopramide prior to infusion, while 2 had received metoclopramide by continuous infusion as the first type of metoclopramide treatment.

    In 2 hospitals we compared the patient charges for
metoclopramide by conventional intermittent bolus
administration with the patient charges for the
metoclopramide by infusion. The bolus charge in each
hospital was considered to be 100 percent. In each
hospital, the cost of metoclopramide to the hospital was
approximately equal. Differences in cost between the
hospitals and between bolus and infusion were due to
charges for admixture of the metoclopramide and for the
other solutions given with metoclopramide. In hospital A,
the infusion charge was only 27 percent of the bolus
charge. In hospital B, the infusion charge was 75 percent
of the bolus charge.

CONCLUSIONS

    We conclude that metoclopramide administered by a
loading dose followed by continuous infusion has only
infrequent side effects but a high frequency of
effectiveness in palliation of chemotherapy associated
vomiting. Metoclopramide infusion is usually preferred by
patients compared to metoclopramide by conventional bolus
injection. We recommend a dose of metoclopramide of 3
milligrams per kilogram administered over 15 minutes as a
loading dose, followed by a continuous infusion of 0.4
milligrams per kilogram per hour for 10 to 24 hours,
depending upon the duration of chemotherapy administration.
Lastly, we have found that metoclopramide infusion is in 2
hospitals less expensive by a variable amount than
metoclopramide bolus injection.

REFERENCES

Taylor WB, Proctor SJ, Bateman DN (1984).
Pharmacohimetics and efficacy of high dose metoclopramide
given by intravenous infusion for the control of cytotoxic
drug induced vomiting.
Br. J. Clin. Pharmacol. 18: 679-684.

Advances in Cancer Control: The War on Cancer—
15 Years of Progress, pages 303–312
© 1987 Alan R. Liss, Inc.

CONTINUOUS INFUSION METOCLOPRAMIDE: CLINICAL TRIALS,
PHARMACOKINETIC CONSIDERATIONS AND COST-EFFECTIVENESS

Peter J. Parashos, William M. Dugan, Jr., Michael
W. Fry
Cancer Center (P.J.P., W.M.D.), School of Pharmacy
and Pharmacal Sciences (M.W.F.)
Methodist Hospital of Indiana, Inc., Indianapolis,
Indiana. 46202. Purdue University, West Lafayette,
Indiana 47907.

INTRODUCTION

The technological advances in cancer research have
resulted in aggressive and innovative chemotherapeutic
regimens and a corresponding increase in drugs with
significant emetogenic potential. Cisplatin, a highly versatile
and widely used antineoplastic agent, in high therapeutic
doses has been reported to result in nausea and vomiting in
nearly 100% of the patients treated.

Numerous antiemetic protocols have been developed for
the prevention of cisplatin-induced nausea and vomiting
(Wampler, 1983). The most encouraging results come from
studies using metoclopramide in combination with other agents
also possessing antiemetic activity. Dexamethasone, shown
to be significantly superior to placebo for the control of
nausea and emesis (Cassileth et al., 1983), (Rhinehart et al.,
1986), diphenhydramine, which also has antiemetic activity
attributable to its antihistamine activity (Physician's
Desk Reference, 1986) and metoclopramide in combination
demonstrated a 93% major response (0-2 vomiting episodes),
(Kris et al., 1985).

The use of multiple intravenous infusions of metoclopramide
in controlling cisplatin-induced emesis has gained widespread
acceptance in oncology practice. Metoclopramide doses of
2mg/ kg at 30 minutes prior to starting cisplatin therapy
and the 1.5, 3.5, 5.5 and 8.5 hours after it's initiation has
become the standard (Gralla et al., 1981).

Graph 1 below illustrates the pharmacokinetic profile of multiple intravenous infusions of metoclopramide given at 2mg / kg for 5 doses as described above.

Multiple Intravenous Infusions of Metoclopramide 2mg/kg x 5 Doses

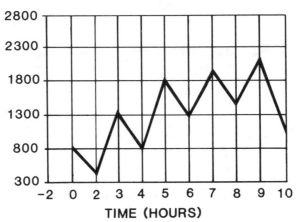

METOCLOPRAMIDE (Ng/MI)

TIME (HOURS)

* Adapted from Taylor W.B., Bateman D.N. High Dose Metoclopramide-Preliminary Pharmacokinetic Studies. Br J. Clin Pharmac. 1983;16:341.

We conducted a pilot study using metoclopramide 2mg/kg IV every four hours for 5 total doses in adult patients scheduled to receive cisplatin in the 60-75mg/m^2 range. Blood samples were drawn 15 minutes after the fifth metoclopramide dose.

Patient	Metoclopramide Blood Level (ng/ml)
1	1528
2	2063
3	1275
4	2705
5	1370
6	1469
7	1900
8	1154
9	1234

Patient	Metoclopramide Blood Level (ng/ml)
10	822
11	679
12	1536
13	1145
14	1268
15	722
16	859
17	1200
18	730

$$\overline{X} = 1317 \text{ ng/ml}$$

The data above shows the mean peak metoclopramide level is less than the theoretical 2000 ng/ml. This is in part due to the wider dosage interval of four hours versus the standard two hour interval discussed earlier. Furthermore, there exists a wide range in peak levels (679-2705 ng/ml) indicating large interpatient variability in drug clearance. Considering this variability in drug clearance, an every four hour interval may result in a subtherapeutic response. This may necessitate a two to three hour dosage interval when using high doses of metoclopramide to prevent cisplatin-induced emesis (Meyer, 1984).

Although these regimens are highly effective in controlling cisplatin-induced emesis, especially when used in combination with diphenhydramine and dexamethasone, they have the major disadvantages of being both costly and cumbersome to the patient and health care provider. It would appear that multiple benefits can be derived by administering metoclopramide as a loading dose followed by a continuous maintenance infusion.

Cost Analysis

Pharmacy Fees: Cost of drug, cost of delivery system, labor cost and professional dispensing fees.

Nursing Fees: Drug administration time, charting time and monitoring time.

Antiemetic Regimens: 1. Intermittent Intravenous Dosing
metoclopramide 2mg/kg x 5 doses
diphenhydramine 50 mg x 1
dexamethasone 20 mg x 1

2. Continuous Intravenous Dosing
load: metoclopramide 2.5 mg/kg
maintenance:metoclopramide 0.5mg/kg / hr
diphenhydramine 50 mg x 1
dexamethasone 20 mg

Intermittent versus Continuous

	Intermittent	Continuous	Difference	+ Potential savings per 750 pts
*Drug	166	110	56	42,000
**Pharmacy Labor	12.25	6.85	5.40	4,050
***Nursing Labor	169	102	67	50,250
				96,300
		less cost of IV pump		−18,750
				$77,550

*Based on average wholesale price 1986

**Extensive time and motion studies in actual hospital pharmacy settings. American Society of Hospital Pharmacists. Dallas, Texas. 1984.

***An application and adaptation of the GRASP Nursing Work-load Management System 1981.

+ Annual number of patients receiving cisplatin at Methodist Hospital of Indiana, Inc., Indianapolis, IN 46202. 1985.

Continuous Infusion

Pharmacokinetic considerations. Graph 2 below illustrates the pharmacokinetic basis of administering metoclopramide as a continuous maintenance infusion.

CONTINUOUS INFUSION

Pharmacokinetic Considerations

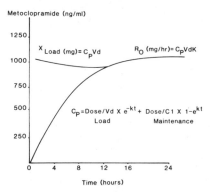

Metoclopramide (ng/ml)

X Load (mg)$= C_p Vd$ R_O (mg/hr)$= C_p VdK$

$C_p = $Dose/Vd X e^{-kt} + Dose/C1 X $1-e^{kt}$
Load   Maintenance

Time (hours)

May need to be altered based on :
1) Cisplatin dose
2) Cisplatin Infusion Time
3) Antineoplastic Agents with delayed onset of emesis

Cp = concentration in the plasma
Vd = volume of distribution
Ro = zero order infusion rate
K = elimination rate constant
+ = infusion time

Clinical Trials

Adult patients below were given metoclopramide 2.5 mg/kg IV follow by a continuous intravenous infusion at 0.5 mg/kg/hr hr. Diphenhydramine 50 mg IV and Dexamethasone 20 mg IV were given as adjunctive antiemetic agents. Patients 1-6 were given metoclopramide as a 12 hour maintenance infusion. Those patients receiving cyclophosphamide (7-11) as part of their chemotherapeutic regimen, had their infusions extended to 18 hours due to it's delayed onset of emesis (Fetting, 1982). Blood samples were drawn at either 11 hours (patient 1-6) or 17 hours (patients 7-11) after starting the maintenance infusion and analyzed for metoclopramide.

Patient	Chemotherapy	Metoclopramide (ng/ml)	Emesis
1	cisplatin 75mg/m^2 etoposide 100mg/m^2	1138	1
2	cisplatin 75mg/m^2 methotrexate 25mg/m^2 5 FU 500 mg/m^2	1600	0
3	cisplatin 60mg/m^2 methotrexate 25mg/m^2 5 FU 500mg/m2	1433	1
4	cisplatin 65mg/m^2 5 FU 500mg/m^2	1469	3
5	cisplatin 75mg/m^2 etoposide 100mg/m^2	1054	0
6	cisplatin 60mg/m^2 5 FU 500mg/m^2	1707	4
7	cisplatin 60mg/m2 doxorubicin 30mg/m^2 cyclophosphamide 500mg/m2	1460	1
8	cisplatin 60mg/m^2 doxorubicin 30mg/m^2 cyclophosphamide 500mg/m2	1308	10+
9	cisplatin 60mg/m2 doxorubicin 30mg/m2 cyclophosphamide 500mg/m^2	1258	1
10	cisplatin 60mg/m2 doxorubicin 50mg/m^2 cyclophosphamide 500mg/m2	1297	0
11	cisplatin 50 mg/m^2 doxorubicin 50mg/m^2 cyclophosphamide 500mg/m2	1101	1

The patients above were all adults (ranging in age from 29-72) with a Karnofsky performance level of 50 or greater.

All patients were in their third cycle of chemotherapy with cisplatin. The mean emetic response for patients 1-6 was 1.5. Whereas the mean emetic response for patients 7-11 was 2.6, and if patient 8 is excluded, 0.5. None of the patients did worse on this regimen than with the first two antiemetic treatments which involved intermittent intravenous dosing with metoclopramide.

For those patients receiving cisplatin as a 5 day continuous infusion (Salem, 1984), we used the following metoclopramide regimen.

Cisplatin 20mg/m^2
5 Day Treatment
Metoclopramide Regimen

Load	Maintenance	Total Dose (mg)
Day 1 2mg/kg	0.4mg/kg/hr x 8 hours	364
Day 2 1.75mg/kg	0.34mg/kg/hr x 8 hours	313
Day 3 1.5mg/kg	0.27mg/kg/hr x 8 hours	256
Day 4 1.2mg/kg	0.23mg/kg/hr x 7 hours	197
Day 5 1.0mg/kg	0.18mg/kg/hr x 5 hours	133

Adjunctive Antiemetics
dexamethasone 4-12mg
diphenhydramine 25-50mg
lorazepam 1-6mg

The dose of metoclopramide is reduced by approximately 50mg per day in the patient weighing 70kg. Dexamethasone, if used for greater than two days is reserved for those patients who have subtherapeutic antiemetic response with the existing treatment or in those patients who develop diarrhea. Diphenhydramine is used once daily prior to initiating metoclopramide therapy. Lorazepam may also be used for prophylaxis of extrapyramidal side-effects and also for its amnestic properties. Although some patients may eventually require no antiemetics at all with this dose of cisplatin generally on the first treatment we will use this approach and treat moderately aggressive to ensure that their initial experience with chemotherapy is positive.

Triple Antiemetic Admixture System
We investigated the possibility of administering dexamethasone and diphenhydramine as a continuous intravenous infusion with metoclopramide in a single carrier solution.

	Load	Maintenance
metoclopramide	2.5 mg/kg	0.5mg/kg/hr
dexamethasone	0.12mg/kg	0.03mg/kg/hr
diphenhydramine	0.5mg/kg	0.05mg/kg/hr

Example:
70 kg patient with adenocarcinoma of the colon. Chemotherapy cisplatin 60mg/m^2, 5 FU 500mg/m^2.
Load: metoclopramide 2.5mg/kg   175mg
       dexamethasone 0.12mg/kg   8mg
       diphenhydramine 0.5mg/kg   35mg
Administered in 100mls of D5W or NS IV over 15 minutes.
Maintenance: metoclopramide 0.5mg/kg/hr   350mg
             dexamethasone 0.03mg/kg/hr   21mg
             diphenhydramine 0.05mg/kg/hr   35mg
Administered in 500mls D51/2 NS IV over 10 hours

A) Physical properties
        Reglan (R), Benadryl (B), Dexamethasone (D)
        *R + B
        *R + D
        B + D yields precipitate.

*Package Insert. Reglan, A.H. Robins. Richmond, VA. Add 3mls of sterile water, D5W or normal saline-precipitate disappears.

B) Chemical properties
    The intent of this study was to show data which would suggest the chemical stability of a triple mixture of diphenhydramine, dexamethasone and metoclopramide in normal saline.

    A triple mixture of the three agents was prepared in the concentrations and conditions shown below and evaluated using high pressure liquid chromatography

*Drugs	Concentrations
Reglan	1.5mg/ml
Benadryl	1.0mg/ml
Dexamethasone	0.5mg/ml

Conditions: The three drugs combined in concentrations described above tested in normal saline only, stored room temperature (25° C) and protected from light. Samples were drawn at 0, 6, 12, 18 and 24 hours after mixing.

*Reglan 50mg/10ml. A.H. Robins. Lot 842379
Benadryl 50mg/ml. Parke-Davis. Lot 01654P
Dexamethasone sodium phosphate 4mg/ml. Elkins-Sinn.
Lot 035177

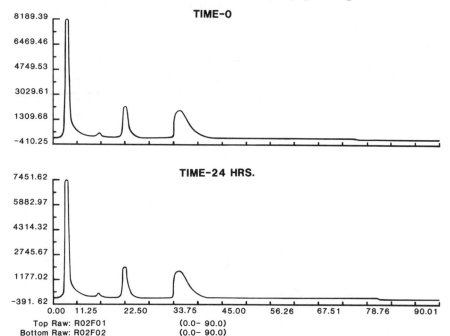

High Pressure Liquid Chromatography Analysis

Conclusions

1. Well designed studies using metoclopramide are further needed to compare it's antiemetic benefit when administered as intermittent intravenous infusions versus continuous drug administration.

2. Until single agent therapy is forwarded, most patients who are treated with cisplatin will receive high doses of metoclopramide, with any one or combination of dexamethasone, diphenhydramine or lorazepam.

3. Continuous infusion metoclopramide is both practical and simple and provides antiemetic and economic benefit in patients treated with cisplatin in the 50-80 mg/m^2 range in combination chemotherapy regimens.

4. Preliminary data indicates that the antiemetic agents, at the concentrations tested, are compatible in normal saline solution for 24 hours at room temperature and when protected from light.

REFERENCES

Cassileth PA, Lusk EJ, Torri S, DiNubile N, Gerson SL (1983).
Antiemetic efficacy of dexamethasone therapy in patients
receiving cancer chemotherapy. Arch Intern Med. 143: 1347–
1349.

Fetting JH, McCarthy LE, Borison HL, Colvin M (1982).
Cyclophosphamide and phosphoramide mustard induced vomiting
in cats. 66:1625–1629.

Gralla RJ, Itri LM, Pisko SE, Squillante AE, Kelsen DP,
Braun DW, Jr., Bordin LA, Braun TJ, Young CW (1981).
Antiemetic efficacy of high dose metoclopramide: Randomized
trials with placebo and prochlorperazine in patients with
chemotherpay-induced nausea and vomiting. N Engl J. Med.
305:905–909.

Kris MG, Gralla RJ, Tyson LB, Clark RA, Kelsen DP, Reilly LK,
Groshen S, Bosl GL, Kalman LA (1985). Improved control of
cisplatin-induced emesis with high-dose metoclopramide and
with combinations of metoclopramide, dexamethasone and
diphenhydramine. Cancer 55:527–534.

Meyer BR, Lewin M, Drayer DE, Pasmantier M, Lonski L,
Reidenberg MM (1984). Metoclopramide control of cisplatin-
induced emesis. Ann Inter Med. 100:393–395.

Rhinehart SN, Dugan WM, Jr., Parashos PJ, Triplett WC (1986).
The added value of dexamethasone to combination drug therapy
in the prevention of cisplatin-induced nausea and vomiting
evaluated by time-lapse video technology. Advances in
Cancer Control. New York: Alan R. Liss, pp. 407–416.

Salem P, Khalyl M, Jabboury K. Cis-Diamminedichloroplatinum
(11) by 5 day continuous infusion. (1984). Cancer 53:
837–840.

Wampler G (1983). The pharmacology and clinical effectiveness
of phenothiazines and related drugs for managing chemo -
therapy-induced emesis. Drugs. 25 (Suppl 1): 35–51.

Advances in Cancer Control: The War on Cancer—
15 Years of Progress, pages 313–320
© 1987 Alan R. Liss, Inc.

IN SEARCH OF NEW CANCER CHEMOPREVENTATIVE AGENTS

Michael J. Wargovich

Section of Gastrointestinal Oncology and
Digestive Diseases, M.D. Anderson Hospital
and Tumor Institute, University of Texas
System Cancer Center, Houston, Texas
77030

INTRODUCTION

Gastrointestinal cancer in the 1980's poses a
difficult clinical challenge. Malignancies of the
gastrointestinal tract have proven refractory to
chemotherapeutic and radiotherapeutic palliation.
Often the only recourse is a surgical excision of
the tumor with intensive follow-up. That
gastrointestinal cancer might result from exposure
to carcinogens of dietary origin and accelerated by
imbalances in nutrition is a theory that has gained
acceptance in the research community. Within the
last 10 years much has been gained by the discovery
of dietary carcinogens and only now are the pieces
of the puzzle are being assembled with reference to
dietary cause and effect of human cancers.

More recent evidence has pointed in another
direction. Since striking differences have been
observed in rates for certain populations for
cancer of the colon, it is conjectured that some
foods may contain *anticarcinogenic* substances,
i.e., chemicals that inhibit carcinogenesis or
delay the progression of the disease. For example,
the consumption of green and yellow leafy
vegetables has been linked to lower risk for
several cancers (Hirayama, et al,1979). In terms

of a mechanistic definition, colon carcinogenesis
seems to follow the classical two-step process
described for other organs. Newly discovered
anticarcinogens may exert their effects in one or
both of the two postulated phases : **initiation** and
promotion.

INHIBITORS OF INITIATION

The first experimental clues to the existence
of anticarcinogenic compounds in foods arose from
the observed suppression of tumorigenicity in
animals fed diets composed of selected dried fruits
and vegetables (Boyd, et al, 1982). Further
investigations led to chromatographic separation
and identification of the chemicals responsible for
the observed decrease in tumorigenicity. A partial
list of chemicals that have been shown to inhibit
experimental forms of cancer and their dietary
sources are shown in Table 1.

TABLE 1. Anticarcinogenic Compounds in Food

Chemical	Food Sources	References
Phenolic acids	most vegetables	Newmark, 1984
Indoles	cruciferous vegetables	Wattenberg, et al,1978
Flavonoids	most fruits	Huang, et al, 1983
Thioethers	garlic, onion	Wargovich, in press
Dithiolthiones	cruciferous vegetables	Ansher, et al, 1986
Aromatic iso-thiocyanates	cruciferous vegetables	Wattenberg, 1977
Tocopherols	nuts, seeds	Mergens, 1978

Inhibitors of initiation are thought to act by one
of several mechanisms. In the case of plant
phenolic acids such as ellagic acid, a structural

similarity between this compound and polycyclic hydrocarbons allows for nucleophilic reaction with the carcinogen (Wood, et al, 1982). Ellagic acid, found in apples and grapes, inhibits lung and skin tumors in the mouse induced by benzo[a]pyrene (Lesca, 1983; Muktar, et al, 1986). Inhibition of cancer by alterations in enzymes responsible for carcinogen metabolism is the postulated mechanism of action for a number of dietary anticarcinogens including flavonoids, dithiolthiones, indoles, and isothiocyanates. Again, a specificity for polycyclic hydrocarbons has prevailed in these studies, most likely to be related to similar metabolic pathways of activation. Specific induction of carcinogen detoxification enzymes such as glutathione transferase has been reported in mice following consumption of diets containing soya bean, Brussels sprouts, cauliflower, alfalfa, or onion (Bradfield, et al, 1985), as well as purified dietary chemicals. For instance, dithiolthiones found in cabbage strongly induce glutathione transferase leading to biochemical detoxification of the carcinogen. Lastly, prevention of carcinogen formation by the antioxidant properties of ascorbic acid and tocopherol (Mergens, et al, 1978) have been demonstrated.

Studies in our laboratory have focused on the unique biochemistry and pharmacology of organic sulfides found naturally in the garlic and onion. In many cases the thioethers found in these herbs are responsible for the characteristic odor and taste of these vegetables. We have investigated the thioether, diallyl sulfide (DAS), a flavor component of garlic, for the ability to inhibit experimentally induced cancer of the colon. DAS had been previously shown by us to inhibit DNA damaging activity by the carcinogen, dimethylhydrazine (Wargovich and Goldberg, 1985). We found strong inhibition of the carcinogenic damage in proliferating cells of the colon when DAS was given 3h prior to the carcinogen. When DAS was tested in animals in a colon tumorigenesis assay it inhibited the incidence of colon cancer by 75%. This result is important in a number of respects. First, we report that a naturally occurring sulfide inhibited the effects of a *methylating* carcinogen (DMH) that is structurally unrelated to polycyclic aromatic hydrocarbons; methylating carcinogens are the most successful agents used to induce gastrointestinal cancer. Secondly, protection by DAS is conferred rapidly once administered. In our tumorigenesis study DAS was also given 3h prior to the carcinogen.

What are the prospects for clinical testing of dietary anticarcinogens? The answer will come after the necessary mechanistic studies to determine efficacy of use in humans and the determination of safety of use of these new agents in purified form.

INHIBITORS OF TUMOR PROMOTION

The process of tumor promotion in gastrointestinal cancer is as yet nearly impossible to define accurately but certain features are known. Many dietary components have been shown to "promote" gastrointestinal cancer, including differing sources and concentrations of fat and fiber, salt, or micronutrients (National Academy of Sciences, 1982). Analysis of results is confounded by the problems of life-time feeding of the putative promoter even during administration of the carcinogen (Reddy and Maeura, 1984). In the purest sense these experiments can not be defined in terms of promotion, but as co-carcinogenesis. Still, a commonalty emerges from these experiments: enhanced cellular proliferation is a generalized feature of tumor promotion of gastrointestinal cancer. Agents that have been reported to increase proliferation of mucosal cells at various sites of the gastrointestinal tract are shown in Table 2.

Table 2. Dietary Agents that Enhance
Gastrointestinal Cancer and Cellular
Proliferation

Organ Site	Dietary Compound	Reference
Esophagus	zinc deficiency	Barch & Iannoccone, 1986
Stomach	salt	Takahashi, et al, 1984
Colon	lipids; wheat bran	Bird & Stamp, 1986; Lupton & Jacobs, 1986

The question of inhibition of tumor promotion
remains difficult because of the complexity of the
biochemical events yet unidentified that lead the
initiated cell to become malignant. One avenue of
approach is to interdict the agents that enhance
cellular proliferation. These compounds in a sense
may be considered *antipromoters*. In our laboratory
we have investigated the mechanism by which dietary
lipids, viz., secondary bile acids and fatty acids
(the predominant chemical forms of fat in the
colon) cause cellular damage and subsequent
proliferation.

Under conditions of basic pH dietary bile
acids and fatty acids are highly ionized and
capable of injuring the mucosa (Wargovich, et al,
1983). Ionized lipids exhibit detergent-like
behavior and are avid scavengers of monovalent and
divalent cations. Therefore excess lipid in the
colonic lumen could sequester mucosal calcium. The
crux of the calcium hypothesis suggested by
Newmark, et al, (1986) is that maintenance of
mucosal calcium levels are vital for a number of
reasons. First, calcium is required for integrity
of intracellular tight junctions; loss of calcium
causes epitheliolysis that may be a signal for
induction of proliferation. Secondly, calcium is
important intracellularly in the regulation of
cellular mitosis and DNA synthesis through a

process mediated by the calcium binding protein, calmodulin (Hait and Lazo, 1986). We have found that sufficient dietary calcium could offset the debilitating effects of ionized bile or fatty acids in studies in mice (Wargovich, et al, 1984) In human studies the calcium hypothesis has found support in a cohort study and in a small clinical trial involving calcium supplementation to patients at high risk for colon cancer (Lipkin and Newmark, 1985).

THE SEARCH CONTINUES

Obviously the discovery of naturally occurring chemicals that may prevent human cancer has created an extraordinary opportunity for future research. Almost certainly, combined modalities of anticarcinogens and antipromoters will be tested for the potential to inhibit the gastrointestinal carcinogenesis. We are considering the possibility of using organic sulfides and calcium tandemly in animals to inhibit esophageal and colon cancer. It is hoped that studies of this nature will serve to pioneer other attempts to thwart the cancer process by natural means.

ACKNOWLEDGEMENTS

The work described here has been supported in part from grants from the Elsa U. Pardee Foundation, the National Dairy Promotion and Research Board in cooperation with the National Dairy Council, and by the University of Texas Cancer Center.

REFERENCES

Ansher SS, Dolan P, and Bueding E (1986). Biochemical effects of dithiolthiones. Fd Chem Toxicol 24(5):405-415.
Barch D and Iannaccone P (1986). Role of zinc deficiency in carcinogenesis. In: "Symposium on Role of Essential Nutrients in Carcinogenesis", Plenum Press, New York.

Bird RP and Stamp D (1986). Effect of a high fat diet on the proliferative indices of murine colonic epithelium. Cancer Lett 33:61-67.

Boyd JN, Babish JG, Stoewsand GS 1982. Modification by beet and cabbage diets of alflatoxin B_1-induced rat plasma -fetoprotein elevation, hepatic tumorignesis, and mutagenicity of urine. Fd Chem Toxicol 20:47-51.

Bradfield CA, Chang Y, Bjeldanes LF (1985). Effects of commonly consumed vegetables on hepatic xenobiotic-metabolizing enzymes in the mouse. Fd Chem Toxicol 23(10) 899-904.

Hait WN, Lazo JA (1986). Calmodulin: A potential target for cancer chemotherapeutic agents. J Clin Oncol 4:994-1012.

Hirayama T (1979). Diet and cancer. Nutr Cancer 1:67-81.

Huang MT, Wood AW, Newmark HL, Sayer JM, Yagi H, Jerina DM, Conney AH (1983). Inhibition of the mutagenicity of bay region diol epoxides of polycyclic aromatic hydrocarbons by phenolic plant flavonoids. Carcinogenesis 4(12) 1631-1637.

Lesca P (1983). Protective effects of ellagic acid and other plant phenols on benzo(a)pyrene induced neoplasia in mice. Carcinogenesis 4(12) 1651-1653.

Lupton J, Jacobs L (1986). Relationship between colonic luminal pH, cell proliferation, and colon carcinogenesis in 1,2-dimethylhydrazine treated rats fed high fiber diets. Cancer Res 46:1727-1734.

Mergens WJ, Kamm JJ, Newark HL, Fiddler W, Pensabene J (1978). Alpha tocopherol: Uses in preventing nitrosamine formation. In: Environmental Aspects of N-Nitroso Compounds, IARC Scientific Publ #119, pp 199-212, IARC, Lyon.

Muktar H, Das M, Bickers D (1986). Inhibition of 3-methylcholanthrene induced skin tumorigenicity in BALB/c mice by oral feeding of trace amounts of ellagic acid in drinking water. Cancer Res 46:2262-2265.

Newmark HL, Wargovich MJ, Bruce WR (1984).   Colon
    cancer and dietary fat, phosphate, and calcium:
    a hypothesis.   JNCI 72:1323-1325.
Reddy BS, Maeura Y (1984).   Tumor promotion by
    dietary fat in azoxymethane-induced colon
    carcinogenesis in female F344 rats: Influence
    of amount and source of dietary fat.   JNCI
    72:745-750.
Takahashi M, Takeshi K, Furukawa F, Kurokawa Y,
    Itayashi Y (1984).   Effects of sodium chloride,
    saccharin, phenobarbital, and aspirin on
    gastric carcinogenesis in rats after initiation
    with n-methyl-n-nitro-n-nitrosoguanidine.   Gann
    75:494-501.
Wargovich MJ, Eng, VWS, Newmark HL, Bruce WR
    (1983).   Calcium ameliorates the toxic effect
    of deoxycholic acid on colonic epithelium.
    Carcinogenesis 4(9) 1205-1207.
Wargovich MJ, Eng VWS, Newmark HL (1984).   Calcium
    inhibits the damaging and compensatory
    proliferative effects of fatty acids on colonic
    epithelium.   Cancer Lett 23:253-258.
Wargovich MJ.   Diallyl sulfide - a flavor
    component of garlic [Allium sativum] inhibits
    dimethylhydrazine induced colon cancer.   (in
    press)
Wattenberg LW, Loub WD (1978).   Inhibition of
    polycyclic hydrocarbon-induced neoplasia by
    naturally occurring indoles.   Cancer Res
    38:1410-1413.
Wattenberg LW (1972).   Inhibition of carcinogenic
    effects of polycyclic hydrocarbons by benzyl
    isothiocyanate and related compounds.   JNCI
    58:395-398.

Index

321